Rural health care

Issues and problems in health care

Paul R. Torrens, M.D., M.P.H., Series editor

School of Public Health,
University of California,
Los Angeles

Rural health care

Milton I. Roemer, M.D.

Professor of Public Health,
University of California,
Los Angeles

Saint Louis

The C. V. Mosby Company

1976

Printed in the United States of America

Distributed in Great Britain by Henry Kimpton, London

Library of Congress Cataloging in Publication Data

Roemer, Milton Irwin, 1916-
 Rural health care.

 (Issues and problems in health care)
 Bibliography: p.
 1. Rural health services—United States—Addresses,
essays, lectures. 2. Rural health services—Addresses,
essays, lectures. I. Title.
RA445.R73   362.1'0973   76-6880
ISBN 0-8016-4166-7

TS/M/M 9 8 7 6 5 4 3 2 1

Preface

While the United States has become increasingly urbanized, the rural population has by no means dwindled away. Definitions of "rural" have changed over the years, but without examining the technicalities, the rural proportion of the U.S. population declined from 54.3% in 1910 to 26.5% in 1970. In numbers of persons, however, because of the overall growth of the national population, this meant a rise from 49,973,000 to 53,886,000 people living in places of under 2500 residents. Applying the definition of rural as meaning the population living outside "metropolitan areas" (cities of 50,000 or more plus all the counties contiguous to the ones containing such cities), the nonmetropolitan population in 1970 was 31.4% of the total or 63,798,000 people.

Thus, by either definition, the rural population requiring health services in America is sizable—greater than that of the entire United States in 1880 (50,156,000). Thanks mainly to greatly improved transportation, the accessibility of these millions of people to health services has markedly improved, but many millions still face handicaps of rural location and rural life. Because of these handicaps, a variety of special efforts have been undertaken to improve the availability of preventive and curative services to rural Americans.

This volume presents five papers analyzing the problem of rural health services along several dimensions. Starting with a nationwide view, it explores the historical development of organized social efforts to tackle rural health problems, which can be traced at least from the period of the Civil War to the present. Chapter 2 focuses on one rural county and on the history of one crucial health sector, that of the public health movement. In Chapter 3 the diversity of organized health programs identified and analyzed in a single county in 1952 is presented, illustrating the pluralism that is so characteristic of the American health care system, urban or rural.

In Chapter 4 the nationwide status of rural health problems and attempted solutions, as of 1968, is summarized; while the focus is principally on the rural poor, the overview is intended to cast light on the situation in which all 50,000,000 or more rural people find themselves. Chapter 5 takes a glimpse at what other nations have attempted to do to overcome the obstacles of rurality for achieving a reasonable distribution of health manpower, facilities, and services—difficulties faced in virtually all countries from the poorest to the richest. Finally, in the epilogue some recent developments relevant for improved rural health services will be noted.

Although each chapter of this book has been published previously, most of these publications are not easily accessible. It is hoped, therefore, that this collection of papers in one place may provide a convenient reference for anyone interested in the special health problems and programs of rural areas.

In the introduction to each chapter the source is indicated. To the several agencies or publishers concerned, my appreciation is extended for permission to reproduce these materials. The bibliographic references at the ends of the chapters may be helpful to the reader who wishes to pursue further special aspects of this subject.

Rurality, of course, is in some ways a matter of degree; however, as long as medical and sanitary science depend on technological developments linked inevitably to urbanization, we may expect that rural health service support and delivery will long remain a special challenge.

Milton I. Roemer

Contents

5 Rural health care solutions attempted around the world, 108

Epilogue, 119

Rural health care

CHAPTER 1 **Historical perspective on rural health services in America**

Since at least as far back as the U.S. Civil War, the special health deficiencies of America's rural population have been recognized. After about 1900, organized health service programs that focused on correcting these deficiencies began to be launched.

These programs have involved social actions in many spheres: (1) the organized prevention of disease, communicable and other; (2) efforts to improve the distribution of physicians and allied health manpower emanating from several governmental levels and from voluntary efforts; (3) the construction of health facilities with federal subsidies and special priorities for rural areas; (4) programs for particularly disadvantaged rural groups, such as migratory farm workers or American Indians; (5) efforts to improve and maintain the quality of medical care in rural districts; (6) measures to increase the economic accessibility of care; and (7) the movement to strengthen overall health service planning.

This chapter traces the development of these several concurrent efforts. It was prepared for a 1973 federal symposium on "Rural Health Delivery Systems" in Denver, Colorado (subsequently cancelled for lack of funds). This paper is being published simultaneously in Hassinger, E. W., and Whiting, L. R., of the North Central Regional Center for Rural Development: Rural health services: organization, delivery, and use, Ames, Iowa, 1976, Iowa State University Press, pp. 3-25.

A s the United States has become increasingly urbanized, the quality of life of the people "left behind" in the rural areas has become a matter of national concern. Included in that quality is the availability of health service. This paper will attempt to review the organized social actions to provide or improve health services for rural people that have been taken in America since 1900, when this began to be perceived as a special problem. These social actions with health objectives have followed numerous paths, have emanated from both governmental and private initiative, have originated at local, state, and national levels, and have been interwoven with the larger sociopolitical trends of our society. In the brief space available, some oversimplification will be inevitable, but my attempt will be to identify the highlights and clarify the general character of the trends.

Early identification of special rural health needs

The notion that rural life has its health handicaps, in spite of fresh air and sunshine, was expressed as early as 1862 in the First Report of the Commissioner of Agriculture to President Abraham Lincoln.[1, 2] Dr. W. W. Hall described in that report the high incidence of insanity and respiratory disease among farm people, the hazards of miasms around farm houses, gastrointestinal problems associated with the use of outdoor privies, and the longevity of farmers, which he said, "is not so great as we might suppose." Definite statistical evidence of rural morbidity rates did not accumulate until some years later. Mortality in rural populations, age-adjusted, was lower than urban mortality in 1900, and while the differential has declined, it is still probably true. However, the needs of health service have never been defined by death rates alone.[3] Social actions have been stimulated by the problems of disease, pain, suffering, and disability and by the concept of applying medical science to human welfare, regardless of mortality tables.

After the Civil War, America developed rapidly with the expansion to the West, the rise of industry, and the growth of large cities. Thousands of immigrants came from Europe, providing a work force for the factories and, with weak social programs, becoming congested in urban slums. In this atmosphere the prominent issue in health service was to prevent the spread of communicable disease in the cities through better environmental sanitation; later, with the rise of bacteriology, immunizations were developed, along with more standardized policies on isolation and quarantine. The public health movement, which took shape in those years, was essentially urban. The classicial Shattuck Report of 1850, giving rise 20 years later to the first state health department, in the Commonwealth of Massachusetts, was obviously written from the perspective of Boston.[4]

It was not until 1910 that the first health departments, for systematic promotion of preventive service, were organized on a county rather than a city basis; even these units in Kentucky, North Carolina, and Washington were largely oriented to the main towns within the county borders. It was in Robeson County, South Carolina in 1912 that the first local health department with a full-time health officer was established in a county that contained no incorporated place of 2500 or more.[5] After 1909 the work of the Rockefeller Sanitary Commission, which tackled hookworm infestation in Southern counties, underscored the need for proper excreta disposal on farms as well as in city tenements.[6]

Official legal action, in the way of sanitary ordinances, had been taken somewhat earlier. In a study of one rural county of West Virginia, I found that a county board of health—with the duty of enforcing various ordinances—had been set up in 1891.[7] The first county health officer, however, was evidently not appointed until 1909, and he was simply a local practicing physician who was assigned certain legal duties. It was not until 1929 that a full-time health officer was appointed and paid to serve the county, with his office all too typically in the basement of the county courthouse.

By the end of World War I the United States had acquired a powerful economic and political position in the world, and several movements for improved health service began to take shape throughout the nation. With the advantage of hindsight, we can identify these movements along several distinct paths—organized disease prevention, health manpower, hospital development, improved financing of medical care, etc. Each of these movements had clear implications for the rural areas, and some of them were specifically focused on rural needs. Rather than examining each year or decade chronologically in the half-century since World War I, it will probably be more meaningful to review the main events in each of these paths of development. Obviously, there were close interrelationships among the parallel paths. Since community action came first in the sphere of disease prevention, this movement will be considered first.

Organized prevention of disease

After 1920, the goal of American public health leadership became the achievement of "coverage" of all the nation's 3070 counties with full-time health departments—that is, public health agencies with a scope wide enough to warrant a full-time director. In 1914 there were fourteen such counties, there were 109 in 1920, and by 1930 the number had increased to 505.[8] This relatively rapid growth was doubtless a reflection of the importance attached in those years to control of the common communicable diseases through both personal preventive and environmental sanitation measures.

The enactment of the Sheppard-Towner Act in 1921 contributed to the strengthening of rural county health departments, by providing federal grants to the states for supporting maternal and child health stations for the first time. The rural birthrate then, as now, was higher than the urban birthrate, and giving immunizations to infants, along with counseling mothers on infant feeding and child-rearing, was obviously a worthy social objective in the small towns and villages.[9] A reflection perhaps of the appreciation of rural public health needs mounting in these years is shown by the fact that in 1925 the American Public Health Association changed the name of its Committee on Municipal Public Health Practice (founded in 1920) to the Committee on Administrative Practice.[10] However, the Sheppard-Towner program of health grants was terminated in 1929 under the conservative era of Herbert Hoover, when the emphasis was on private enterprise and local government.

The massive economic depression that started in late 1929 was a setback for rural as well as urban preventive health efforts. Government attention became focused on relief of those who were destitute. It took the Social Security Act of 1935 to give a new boost to preventive services. While many social leaders had urged a health insurance title in the act, President Roosevelt did not wish to become embroiled in the issue of "socialized medicine," and instead Titles V and VI were included in the act.[11] Title V, in effect, reinstated federal grants to the states for maternal and child health services; Title VI gave grants for all the other types of public health services. Since city governments generally had greater revenue resources of their own, these funds were used in large part to build up preventive programs in the more rural counties. The variable matching formula of these grants yielded relatively greater assistance to the poorer states of the South. They also facilitated the strengthening of most state health departments, whose consultation and standard-setting practices (e.g., state sanitary codes) were probably of greatest relevance to rural areas that lacked strong local public health agencies of their own.

By 1942, after the first 7 years of these federal health grants, over 1800 counties had achieved full-time public health coverage, but there were still 1250 counties, mostly rural, without such protection.[12] Part of the rural problem was the small population base and poverty of many counties. As part of the "postwar planning" that accompanied World War II, therefore, the American Public Health Association proposed a plan for consolidating the public health tasks of several adjacent rural counties into multicounty districts and for merging city and county health departments to achieve nationwide public health coverage through about 1200 units.[13] This general strategy has succeeded in attaining public health agency coverage today in about 80% of the nation's counties and a higher proportion of the rural population.[14]

The scope of public health services has generally widened in the United States to include mental health, chronic disease detection, accident prevention, and other activities beyond communicable disease control, but this broader policy seldom applies to the small health departments in rural districts. Moreover, there are many vacancies among these units in the poorer states, where the salaries of health officers are low.[15] The main foot soldiers of rural public health work are the public health nurses and the sanitarians, who have doubtless played a significant role in the reduction of rural infant mortality and number of rural cases of enteric fevers. The ratio of public health nurses per 100,000 population, nevertheless, is still substantially lower in the more rural states, in spite of the greater drain on their time caused by travel.

Newer preventive programs, in which rural health departments have played a significant role, have included family planning and a wider scope for child health, including some treatment services. In the Southeastern states, with large populations of blacks, birth-control advisory services have been offered by rural health departments longer than elsewhere; the small Catholic constituencies and the rapid growth of black compared with white populations may account for this. The recently funded wider-scope MIC (maternity and infant care) and C & Y (children and youth) health care programs, however, are typically found in the large city slums, where medical schools or medical centers are at hand, and seldom in rural districts. Fluoridation of water supplies to prevent dental caries is another measure dependent on efficient public water systems, seldom found in small towns and not at all, of course, in open-country areas.

Thus while the coverage of rural counties with official public health services has shown great improvement since 1910, the scope of services offered has not been as impressive. The "basic six" of the APHA program of 1945, identified with Dr. Haven Emerson, are still the usual boundaries—communicable disease control, environmental sanitation, maternal and child health preventive services, health education, and two instrumentalities of these: vital statistics and laboratory services. Indeed, even within these boundaries, the impacts have probably been small because of meager manpower resources and the timid leadership of most rural health departments.

Improved distribution of health manpower

Perhaps the most obvious health service deficiency perceived by rural people is a shortage of physicians. Not that this was always so; a physician writing from the rural South in 1843 complained of greater competition than in the New England states because of there being "twice the number of doctors that the community needed."[16] But when the output of physicians was greatly reduced following the Flexner revolution in medical education (1910), and when the smaller number of new graduates began to flock to the cities with their greater wealth, more opportunities for specialization, and many cultural advantages, then the lack of rural physicians as well as other health personnel became a prominent issue.

The first social actions to cope with this problem were taken by small towns themselves. In response to this issue, the New Hampshire Legislature in 1923 enacted a statute that read:

> Towns may at any annual meeting vote to raise such sums of money as they may deem necessary towards support of a resident physician in such towns which, in the absence of such appropriation, would be without the services of such physician.[17]

These tax funds could be used to pay the physician for health services to schoolchildren or to the poor, so as to supplement basic earnings from private practice; sometimes they would be used for a direct subsidy on top of private earnings to reach a guaranteed annual income. Other direct actions by rural communities have included inducements of a rent-free house, an automobile, or ready-made office facilities. Petitions for a physician signed by hundreds of citizens have been launched to offer an enticing welcome.[18] Private industrial firms such as mines, public utilities, or lumber companies in isolated areas secured physicians for their workers and dependents by simply paying them salaries from funds raised through wage deductions or management contributions.

Another approach was attempted in the 1930's by the Commonwealth Fund, which gave fellowships to medical students on the condition that they would practice in a rural location for a certain number of years. The results were discouraging, however; after the period of obligation was finished, nearly all these young physicians left the rural town for a larger city. Nevertheless, the same idea was launched by state governments on a larger scale a little later. In 1942 Virginia passed a law to provide tuition and fellowships for the complete medical education of rural youths, who would agree to return to a rural community designated by the state health department as needing a physician. In the later 1940's, about ten other states, mostly in the South, enacted similar programs.

The financial extent of this rural medical fellowship support, however, has never been very great, and it has fluctuated from year to year. When I wrote to Virginia's State Health Commissioner in 1967 to inquire about the results of 20 years of this effort, he replied:

> It is hard to evaluate the effectiveness of the program. Certainly it has not been a great boon to [medical] practice in the rural areas; on the other hand, it has helped to fill a monetary need for these students.[19]

A proper evaluative study of these state government efforts to attract young physicians to rural areas might well be conducted, but the general evidence of persistently lower physician-population ratios in rural counties suggests that they have not been very successful.

In 1953 a state medical society set out to tackle the problem by giving advice and assistance to rural communities in establishing small private clinics to attract physicians. The Tennessee State Medical Association claimed some success in this approach.[20] A few years later, in 1959, the Sears Roebuck Foundation put greater funds in back of this idea—lending money to small towns, along with free architectural plans, to build modern private medical quarters.[21] A North Carolina observer points out, however, that the purely private entrepreneurial base of this program has led to instability; when the physician decides to move away, the clinic building may be sold to an insurance agent or a beauty shop operator.[22]

For some years, the American Medical Association has provided an "information service" on communities needing physicians, through its Council on Rural Health Services. Since 1948 the AMA has also held a series of "National Conferences on Rural Health" to publicize this and other approaches to the problem.

More fundamental attacks on the rural shortage of physicians have been the many actions, especially since the end of World War II, to increase the total national output of physicians, along with many other types of health workers. As long as the overall supply of health manpower is less than the mounting demand, one must expect that the least attractive areas—whether central city slums or rural districts—will get the leanest pickings. Social actions to increase the nationwide output of all types of health manpower have been taken largely by government, at both state and national levels.

In 1945 there were seventy-seven approved medical schools in the United States, but since then the trend of reduction initiated by the Flexner Report has been reversed, so that there are now about 115. Most of the new schools were established by state governments, all of them with public subsidy. Moreover, most schools, both public and private, have increased their enrollments and numbers of graduates.[23] Still, this increase was not enough to accommodate the expanding need of the nation's hospitals for interns and residents, and matters would have been and would still be much worse if it were not for a large inflow of graduates from foreign medical schools.

The expansion of health manpower education, so important for rural areas, depended on an increasing flow of subsidy from the federal government. In spite of initial opposition to such subsidy by the AMA—for fear of federal domination of the professional schools—the need became so glaring that by the mid-1960's general consensus had been achieved. The National Advisory Commission on Health Manpower, reporting in 1967, advocated not only greatly increased numbers of virtually all types of health personnel, but also increased rationalization of the delivery system, so that "new categories of health professionals" could be effectively used.[24]

Such new categories of medical assistant—dating from the Russian "feldsher" of the 1870's—have always been considered especially relevant for thinly settled rural districts. In the decade of the 1960's, several dozen grant programs were initiated, under the auspices of different federal agencies, to subsidize the training of many types of health manpower.[25] In 1971 a Comprehensive Health Manpower Act achieved integration of several of these federal grant programs. Today we see scores of new training programs for "physician assistants," "Medex" personnel, "nurse practitioners," "pediatric associates," "anesthetic technicians," midwives, and others being developed by universities and hospitals, with encouragement from both the government and the private health professions.

Other countries, like Mexico, Iran, or the Soviet Union, have long used another approach to getting physicians into rural areas—invoking national authority. In Mexico, for example, most medical degrees are awarded by the National University of Mexico, and a condition for that degree has been for the new graduate to spend a period of "social service" in a rural district; recently this was increased from 6 months to 1 year. Iran uses the military conscription laws as a vehicle for getting manpower to outlying areas, through a "Rural Health Service Corps." The Soviet Union has long required a 3-year period of rural service for most, though not all, new medical graduates.[26] While the United States has not gone so far as any of these foreign examples, the "National Health Service Corps," set up under the Emergency Health Personnel Act of 1970, has been perhaps a step in this direction. Under this law, physicians, dentists, nurses, and some other health professionals are brought into a federal program, which, in effect, meets military obligations. Then they are sent to communities of need, mostly rural, where they serve the poor without charge and work with others on a fee basis; sometimes they work in organized health units and sometimes in traditional private offices. Of about 5000 communities estimated to need such assistance, a few hundred have so far been helped.[27]

Improvement of the rural health manpower supply has also been tackled through various indirect approaches. Provision of modern hospitals has been one basic strategy, advanced often as a means of attracting new physicians. Promotion of better medical incomes, through various forms of health insurance—social or voluntary—has been another strategy. Regionalized systems and group medical practice have been other mechanisms to render settlement in a rural community less isolated and more stimulating. These approaches to the rural manpower problem will be considered in other contexts below.

Rural health facilities

The importance of general hospitals for good medical care is too obvious to elaborate, but until about 1930 the initiative and financial resources for their construction were entirely dependent on local effort. This did not apply to hospitals for long-term care of mental disorders or tuberculosis, which have been built by state governments since the late nineteenth century, nor to a special "charity hospital" system for the poor in Louisiana. For day-to-day management of serious illness, however, the community general hospitals of the nation required entirely local initiative, usually by voluntary bodies (religious or nonsectarian) and sometimes by local government, especially in rural counties. This resulted in a severe imbalance of hospital bed-population ratios between urban and rural districts, since the latter have always had weaker economic resources.

In the early 1930's the Commonwealth Fund launched a program to help rural communities build small general hospitals, through a two-thirds subsidy of the cost of construction and equipment.[28] Fourteen hospitals were built under this program, and later other foundations, including the Kellogg Foundation in Michigan and the Duke Endowment in North Carolina, gave other forms of capital assistance to rural hospitals.

It took the great Depression to bring the resources of the federal government to bear on this problem. Under the New Deal's Public Works Administration (PWA) and Work Projects Administration (WPA), assistance was given to the construction or improvement of hundreds of hospitals, although mainly in the larger cities. During World War II the Community Facilities Act also provided federal grants to support hospital construction in congested areas springing up incident to war production or military training.[29] Some of this construction, which also established health centers for housing public health agencies, was in small towns that definitely served rural people.

An overview of nationwide hospital needs, which emphasized the deficiencies of rural areas, was first taken as part of postwar planning during World War II. The leadership of the U.S. Public Health Service in those years was extremely important, especially the imaginative role of Dr. Joseph W. Mountin. He and his colleagues published in 1945 the first national survey of hospital bed supply in relation to population in all the counties of the nation, along

with theoretical proposals for action needed to achieve rural-urban equity.[30]
"Health service areas" were defined in which peripheral (rural), intermediate,
and base hospitals should ideally exist. In tandem with this governmental
work, a voluntary national Commission on Hospital Care was established
in 1944, mainly through the initiative of the American Hospital Association,
aided by private foundations. This body's report, "Hospital Care in the United
States," appeared in 1946.[31]

These studies laid the technical basis for the National Hospital Survey
and Construction (Hill-Burton) Act of 1946. This legislation provided grants
to the states to subsidize hospital construction in areas of greatest need, the
latter to be determined by surveys in each state with design of a state "master
plan."[32] The law and regulations under it required that a ranking of priorities
be established, through which areas of greatest deficiency from the optimal
standard of bed need would get assistance first. Inevitably, this meant that
the maximum aid went to building hospitals in rural districts. It is also
noteworthy that the Hill-Burton Act aided hospitals under both governmental
and voluntary nonprofit sponsorship, in fact, mainly the latter, so that the
public-private partnership concept was being implemented 20 years before
the 1966 law labeled as the "Partnership for Health Act." An important
condition of the grants was that certain standards of hospital design be met
and, furthermore, that every state receiving aid enact a hospital licensure
program to assure continuation of proper hospital maintenance and professional practices.

Largely because of the Hill-Burton program, the hospital resources of rural
America have been greatly improved, both in quantity and quality. Between
1946 and 1966 the disparity in bed-supply between the predominantly rural
and urban states was largely eliminated. In fact, in 1964 the Hill-Burton Act
was amended to give grants for "modernization" of facilities, which was
designed to channel more support into the deteriorating hospitals of the larger
cities. Over the years, the law has been repeatedly amended to adjust to newly
perceived needs for chronic disease facilities, new types of health centers,
research in hospital service, and area-wide planning (i.e., below the level of
the state government).

The trend in hospital use by rural people over the last 30 years has clearly
been upward, but this does not mean hospitalization solely in small-town
hospitals. Improvements in transportation have been a major factor, and many
rural patients, especially those of higher income, bypass the nearby community
hospital to seek more specialized care in a distant urban institution.[33]

The actions taken in particular states to improve the supply and operation
of hospitals serving rural people are too numerous to review. Many of the
state health departments, responsible for the Hill-Burton program and for
implementation of the hospital licensure laws, have given special consultations
to upgrade rural hospitals. Some of the state hospital associations have done

likewise. In the Appalachian states, with special federal assistance under the Appalachian Regional Development Act, hospitals and health centers have been particularly expanded to meet the needs of the low-income mountain people.[34] Perhaps because of the drama of serious illness, the hospital sector of rural health needs has shown striking improvement, and other sectors are now drawing greater attention.

Programs for special rural populations

The United States Department of Agriculture and its cooperating state agencies have long operated programs focused on the welfare of farm families. The Agricultural Extension Services, along with their advice to farmers on crop or livestock practices, have had their various "home demonstration" programs, which include education on nutrition, sanitation, and hygienic habits.

Probably the most remarkable health service program directed specifically at farm families of low income was that of the U.S. Farm Security Administration (FSA) in the 1930's and 1940's.[35] As part of a generalized effort to rehabilitate low-income and economically marginal farm families, the FSA gave low-interest loans for various agricultural production purposes, but along with these they also gave assistance on family living. Among the latter were loans, or sometimes grants, for prepaid membership in small local medical care plans providing physician, hospital, and sometimes dental and drug services. At their peak in 1942 these local health insurance plans served over 600,000 persons in 1100 rural counties. There were also special "experimental rural health programs" in six southern counties, in which low-income farm families who were not regular FSA-borrowers were invited to join relatively more comprehensive prepayment plans, with government subsidies of premiums on a sliding scale in proportion to family income. Another special program in Taos County, New Mexico, established rural health centers, with salaried physicians and nurses giving general ambulatory care. However, the overall FSA approach simply accepted the existing private free choice custom and heightened access to care through prepayment.

With the retrenchment of federal assistance from the U.S. Department of Agriculture after World War II, this program gradually declined, and the health needs of low-income farm families were left to be met by the traditional local welfare departments or through the private sector. The FSA experience, however, doubtless left its mark in a heightened appreciation of the special problems of rural medical care. Farm organizations, like the Farmers Union and the Grange, if not the more big-grower–oriented Farm Bureau, became sensitized to these issues. Enrollment of farm people in Blue Cross and other health insurance plans, the founding of some voluntary rural medical cooperatives, and support for the whole concept of hospital regionalization were probably among the long-term benefits of this experience.

Another special rural population group for which the USDA provided health care were migratory farm workers.[36] Originally one sector of the FSA program, this was shifted during World War II to a special Office of Labor under the War Food Administration. To cope with the special needs of these families who, because they were nonresidents, did not usually qualify for local welfare medical aid, a network of clinics was set up at about 250 locations of seasonal labor concentration around the country. Physicians on part-time salary and full-time nurses with rather broad "standing orders" (shades of the "nurse practitioner" of the 1970's) staffed these clinics. To cut through bureaucratic impediments in hiring personnel, purchasing supplies, and so on, a series of six "Agricultural Workers' Health and Medical Associations"—nonprofit corporations established locally—were organized to take direct responsibility, entirely under federal financial support.

Although this program also died after World War II, the plight of migratory families continued and, as happened for American poverty in general, was "rediscovered" in the early 1960's. In 1962, the federal Migrant Health Act was passed, reestablishing federal aid for health services to migrant workers and their dependents.[37] Instead of direct federal operation or use of quasi-governmental health corporations, however, this program provided grants from the U.S. Public Health Service to state and local agencies—mostly health departments but sometimes local medical societies, religious missions, or other bodies—for services to migrant families. "Family health service clinics," as the law defines them, are the usual modality, although some of the funds have simply been used to strengthen the traditional preventive services of local health departments. Patterns of interstate agricultural migration have obviously changed over the decades, and most seasonal farm labor is now evidently drawn from within state borders, which simplifies the problems of legal entitlement to welfare medical service. Nevertheless, the federal appropriations of a few million dollars for this program have typically been much less than the authorization and far less than the volume of need.

American Indians are an essentially rural ethnic group that has long been the beneficiary of special federal assistance. Of about 700,000 Indians in the nation, approximately half are living in or near reservations entitling them to services from a network of special health centers and hospitals, operated from 1849 to 1955 by the U.S. Department of the Interior, and since then by the U.S. Public Health Service.[38] Most of these facilities are small and staffed by salaried medical and nursing personnel; there are also contractual arrangements with other local hospitals and physicians. The Indian Health Service offers a comprehensive scope of preventive and curative services, putting special stress on problems like tuberculosis and alcoholism, which have high prevalence in this population. While marked progress in increasing life expectancy has been recorded among Indians, their health status is still substantially lower than that of the general population.[39]

A more recent governmental approach to helping special population groups has been that of the U.S. Office of Economic Opportunity (OEO) set up in 1964. With respect to health services, the strategy of the OEO has been to concentrate efforts intensively in certain "pockets of poverty" by establishing "neighborhood health centers," which offer comprehensive ambulatory services to all low-income persons (not solely to public assistance recipients) in the immediate area.[40] These local centers obviously modify traditional patterns of medical care delivery, with their combination of preventive and curative services, a range of salaried medical and surgical specialists, and active "outreach" efforts through community aides to attract the poor into the center for health attention.

The great majority of OEO- supported health centers have been established in central city slums, often in response to urban riots, but a few have been specifically rural, such as the center at King City, California or Mound Bayou, Mississippi. These two units, in fact, as well as many others, have been subjects of sharp controversy associated with local medical opposition and directed at the OEO policy of delegating major administrative responsibilities to the poor people themselves.[41] In spite of these difficulties, the concept of the broad-gauged health service center for ambulatory care was extended throughout the nation under the sponsorship of the U.S. Department of HEW, as well as the OEO. By 1975 all these units were transferred to HEW and designated as "community health centers."

Not all health actions for special rural population groups stem from governmental initiative. The organized efforts of the Welfare and Retirement Fund for coal miners and their families throughout the United States is one of the best examples of voluntary action. While "fringe benefit" health programs resulting from negotiation between labor and management are typically thought of as urban affairs, the coal-mining industry is primarily in rural regions, so these efforts obviously also improve rural health service.

For a century or so, health services in mining or other isolated industries such as lumbering or railroading were developed separately by each local employer.[42] In 1950, after extensive negotiations, the United Mine Workers of America Welfare and Retirement Fund was established through an industry-wide agreement between bituminous coal operators and the union. As a result of the Fund, a wide range of welfare benefits are offered to coal-mining families, including specialist, hospital, and certain high-cost pharmaceutical or long-term services.[43] The general strategy has been to pay for approved services rendered by local physicians and other providers who have been found to meet quality standards. In a number of locations in the coal-mining districts of Appalachia (but also in Pennsylvania, Ohio, and elsewhere), however, the local medical care resources were very deficient, and the Fund stimulated the organization of several new group-practice clinics, with well-qualified specialists. These clinics then served eligible mining families as well as other people in the area. In the late 1950's, the Fund also used its resources to build a network of ten new well-staffed general hospitals in the Appalachian states, where local resources were especially weak.[44] Financial pressures compelled transfer of these in the 1960's to other sponsorship, but all ten hospitals, with relatively strong staffs of full-time specialists, are still in operation serving these rural people.

Quality promotion

Several of the organized health efforts already discussed have, of course, stimulated an improved quality of rural health care, but certain actions, both governmental and voluntary, have been specifically focused on this objective. In my view, the most important of these have been the movements usually epitomized as "regionalization" and "group practice," supplemented by a variety of "regulatory" programs.

The regionalization concept has been mainly directed to assuring rural people the same quality of medical care as is available to people in the cities where highly specialized resources exist. The first systematic program to apply the idea was in the state of Maine in the 1930's, where the Bingham Associates Fund established a series of professional connections between hospitals in the small towns of that state and a large medical center in Boston.[45] There were regular consultation services in pathology, radiology, and other fields, through the mail as well as by visits; the Maine physicians were invited to Boston for postgraduate education; and rural patients with difficult cases were referred to Boston for diagnostic workups or complex therapy. The same concept was implemented in the 1940's in several rural counties around Rochester, New York, also with foundation support.

The Hill-Burton Act, discussed earlier, contemplated cooperative activities among the several echelons of hospitals in a state, following their construction under a regionalized master plan. In practice, however, these interhospital ties did not develop very successfully.[46] The autonomy of both private physicians and sovereign hospitals presented obstacles. Instead of a theoretical two-way flow of patients and consultation services, the most viable programs simply offered educational services from a teaching medical center outward to small community hospitals. After World War II several medical schools undertook such programs.[47]

It took the enactment of Medicare in 1965 to give a substantial boost to the regionalization idea; with all this money being put into paying for services to old people, it was argued, something should be done to underpin the quality of those services. The legislative strategy was to focus attention on the three leading causes of deaths in the nation, especially among the aged—heart disease, cancer, and stroke. In late 1965, therefore, a new federal law was enacted to provide grants for "regional medical programs" (RMP) to deal with the three top killing diseases.[48] Gradually the scope of diseases and also of service modalities under the RMP legislation has widened, and its objectives have evolved toward upgrading the quality of medical care for all conditions in the population living outside the metropolitan centers. In the 1970's special priority is being given to improving the quality of services for the poor, both in large cities and rural districts.

How well the RMP program is promoting the classical concept of regionalization is debatable.[49] Its impact has been primarily educational, and it has done relatively little to encourage regionalized flow of patients or true coordination in the management of hospitals. Still, it has stimulated a number of new services in the smaller hospitals, such as coronary care units, stroke rehabilitation centers, or cancer screening programs. The establishment of various RMP district committees, containing both providers and consumers of health care, has created an additional ferment in the American health service system, which has long-term implications for rural health care. A recently reported personnel exchange program between rural and urban hospitals in the state of Washington is just one illustrative outgrowth of RMP stimulation.[50]

The group practice idea was really pioneered in a rural setting, with the initiative of the Mayo brothers in the small town of Rochester, Minnesota in the 1880's. Opposition to the teaming up of physicians in private clinics, however, was substantial in the urban centers; solo practitioners through the local medical societies looked upon this as unfair competition and often branded it as "unethical." As a result, group medical practice has actually developed more extensively in small towns, where the opposition was weaker, than in large cities. A study in 1959 found 8.2 physicians in group practice clinics per 100,000 population in isolated rural counties, compared with 5.0 per 100,000 in the metropolitan counties.[51]

There are many definitions and forms of group medical practice, but its major import is that a number of physicians and allied health personnel work together and bring to bear many skills on the care of the patient.[52] Since 1965 the growth of group practice in the nation has accelerated, and with the generally high demand for medical care in the population, opposition to this form from solo practitioners has declined. Hospitals have always offered an organized setting in which specialists and allied personnel could work, but the group practice clinic makes this teamwork feasible for the ambulatory patient; it also provides a reasonable economic base for specialists in small towns, where they might not make a satisfactory income working alone.

A few private group practices have taken special initiative to get primary health services out to very isolated rural people. The Rip Van Winkle Clinic in Hudson, New York operated three satellite health stations in outlying villages during the 1950's. The Daniel Boone Clinic in Harlan, Kentucky has two major and three small satellite stations within a forty-mile radius in this depressed mountain area. The Dickenson-Wise Clinic in Wise, Virginia is another rural ambulatory care center with five peripheral branches. Other group practice clinics of distinction, serving mainly rural populations, number in the hundreds and provide centers of quality care for miles around. While the vast majority of these are private and not linked to any prepayment plan, they provide a nucleus for what may later evolve as "health maintenance organizations" (p. 21). Group practices, it should also be noted, are a natural vehicle for attracting new physicians into an area, since there are no problems of setting up a practice; from the first day, the young physician can be busy and useful.

A third stream of quality promotion affecting rural health service are the regulatory activities that usually emanate from a state or higher political level. These are both governmental and voluntary. Beyond the hospital licensure laws, mentioned earlier, there is the Joint Commission on Accreditation of Hospitals (JCAH), founded in 1950.[53] JCAH inspections and approvals may well have more influence on hospitals in rural districts than in cities, since these hospitals are subject to fewer general outside contacts. The Speciality Boards in Medicine, starting with ophthalmology in 1916, have steadily increased their impact. The various professional societies in medicine, dentistry, nursing, etc. exert an influence through continuing education. The American Academy of General Practice requires a certain amount of postgraduate study each year for continued membership of general practitioners, who are of course relatively more numerous in rural areas than in the cities. The most recently established Specialty Board in Family Practice (1969) should help to elevate the status of the general practitioner, and this in turn should result in long-term rural benefits.

Under Medicare every participating hospital must have a "utilization review" process, which induces a certain group discipline in hospital staffs, beyond the usual medical staff rules. In late 1972 federal amendments to the Social Security Act (the Medicare and Medicaid sections) mandated the establishment of Professional Standards Review Organizations (PSRO's) to blanket the nation with medical bodies that would exercise peer review of all hospital cases financed with public funds. These PSRO's when fully implemented should have special significance for the more frequently isolated rural physician and dentist. Another new development is the proposed network of "Area Health Education Centers" (AHEC), designed to provide continuing education for all sorts of health manpower in isolated or low-income regions— evidently to either supplement or replace the RMP activities.

Strengthened economic support

A root problem in attaining good medical care everywhere has always been getting the necessary economic support. For the wealthy this has seldom been an issue, but per capita incomes have long been lower in rural areas, and charity, which has historically helped the poor, is scantier in rural areas. Voluntary health agencies, supported by private donations, are weaker in the more rural states, as reflected in 1966 data from the American Heart Association and the American Cancer Society.[54] The Frontier Nursing Service of Kentucky, supported originally by private philanthropy in the 1920's, is now dependent mainly on governmental grants. Church missions in the Southwest or elsewhere still offer some hospital services, but most of their support comes from noncharitable sources.

Much more important than charity since the 1930's have been the various programs of public assistance, which include support for medical care. Before the Social Security Act of 1935, the welfare programs in rural counties were extremely meager, but the inauguration of federal grants to the states brought definite improvements.[55] Federal assistance is dependent on demographic categories, the largest of which is the program for "Aid to Families with Dependent Children" (AFDC); since children are more numerous in rural families (as well as low-income families generally), this program has special value for rural populations. Over the years the Social Security Act has been amended, widening its medical benefits for the poor. The actual amounts of financial aid, however, are dependent on matching state funds, so the net support per case is typically lower in the more rural than the more urbanized states.

After 30 years of experience, the Social Security Act was amended in 1965 with Title XIX or "Medicaid," which put much larger sums into support of medical care for the poor. In order to qualify for federal grants, states had to assure a relatively wide scope of physician, laboratory, hospital, and extended care services for categorical cash-grant recipients, and also (with limitations) to "medically needy" persons who were categorically linked but not getting cash grants.[56] The various amendments and regulations under the Medicaid programs are too complex to summarize here, but two points should be made: under the program the rural poor have received more medical care than they got before, yet they still receive less care than the urban poor. The reason is not simply the lesser per-person expenditures, but the lower supply of rural physicians and the relative scarcity of hospital outpatient departments, which play such a large part in meeting demands of the urban poor.

The rapidly rising general prices and costs of medical care in the nation since 1965 have created obvious pressures on state governments, which must finance about half of Medicaid costs. This has led to retrenchments of the program in many states, especially with respect to the "medically needy" or the near-poor. A special investigating commission in 1970 recommended federalization of the whole structure of medical care for the poor, and use of public funds for enrolling them in existing health insurance plans serving the general population.[57] Some of the states, like California, are now doing this on a limited basis.

In even the most generous state jurisdictions, only a small percentage of the total population, well under 10%, qualifies for formal public assistance, and the great majority of people must rely on other forms of economic support for medical care. Voluntary health insurance has provided an increasing share of this support over the last 50 years. The early application of the insurance mechanism in isolated industries and the subsidized FSA programs for low-income farm families have been mentioned, but the big national push began with the rise on a community basis of general hospital insurance in 1929, later acquiring the "Blue Cross" emblem. This was supported by the hospitals themselves, and in 1939, state medical societies began to sponsor parallel insurance (Blue Shield) mainly for physician's service in hospitalized cases. In the 1940's the commercial insurance companies, which had previously offered limited indemnity policies for loss of earnings or some medical expenses resulting from accidents or sickness, also began to sell this type of insurance in a big way.[58]

The health insurance movement is too well known to summarize here, but it may simply be noted that its impact on rural, has been much less than on urban populations. The rapid growth of insurance coverage has been caused mainly by enrollment of employed groups, found of course mainly in urban industries. Individual farm families or people in small rural trade centers are not so easily enrolled, even if they can afford it. Thus it was found in 1963 that while about 75% of urban people had some form of insurance protection (usually for hospitalization), this applied to 64% of rural nonfarm people and to only 51% of rural farm people.[59] Moreover, the kind of insurance held by rural people is more often the individual enrollment type of indemnity policy, sold by commercial carriers, which tends to have higher premiums and more restricted benefits (with various exclusions, deductibles, etc.).[60]

Here and there, rural cooperatives that had been organized for agricultural purposes applied the same mechanism to insurance for medical care. One of the first and most illustrious of these efforts was at Elk City, Oklahoma, where the local Farmers Union set up the Farmers Cooperative Health Association in 1929. The struggles of Dr. Michael Shadid to keep this consumer-sponsored program afloat against intense opposition from the state and local medical societies is one of the sagas of hard-won progress in the rural health field.[61] This program, like one developed later at Two Harbors, Minnesota, was associated with salaried group practice and helped to pioneer the principle now heralded nationally as the HMO concept. Most such organizations, however, are confined to city families—particularly the two largest, the Kaiser-Permanente Health Plan and the Health Insurance Plan of Greater New York. This movement has now come to be spearheaded by the Group Health Association of America, but it still reaches only about 5% of the U.S. population, and a smaller percentage of the rural.

Aside from deficiencies in rural health insurance coverage, the prominent gap in the 1950's was the weak insurance protection of aged persons, since after 65 years of age most people are retired from employment. Most private insurance companies, moreover, had specifically excluded older persons from coverage because they are "high risks" (that is, have greater needs for medical care), or else such persons were enrolled only with higher premiums and numerous benefit restrictions. In 1957, therefore, the first federal legislation was proposed to apply social insurance to medical care of the aged, by making hospitalization a supplementary benefit along with old-age pensions under the Social Security Act. This proposal by Representative Aimes Forand generated two responses: an intensive campaign of opposition by the American Medical Association, the insurance industry, and others, mindful of the bitter invectives against the first National Health Bills 15 years earlier. Secondly, it led most of the voluntary insurance plans to expand their benefits for old people, some of which were even mandated by state laws.[62]

Eight years of contention followed, however, before Title XVIII, "Medicare," was added to the Social Security Act in 1965. Workmen's compensation providing medical care for industrial injuries (usually excluding agricultural work, incidentally) had started on a state-by-state basis in 1910, and unsuccessful proposals for state laws to meet the costs of general nonoccupational illness had been debated from 1915 to 1920. Now at last a social insurance law for hospital, physician, and other services—although confined to old people—was enacted for the whole United States. To secure Congressional passage, numerous compromises were made, involving restrictions on benefits associated with commercial insurance practice and day-to-day administration by nongovernmental health plans designated as "fiscal intermediaries."[63] Also, important administrative differences apply to the entitlement of people to hospital and extended care facility services, compared with the services of physicians.

Aged people in rural areas have probably enjoyed the greatest relative improvement from the Medicare law, since their previous insurance coverage was so poor and their socioeconomic status generally so low. One may conjecture that this flow of assured fees has also added appreciably to the income of rural physicians and small-town hospitals. Since aged persons, when hospitalized, have relatively long periods of stay and since their frequency of illness is higher, Medicare payments now account for about 40% of general hospital income and very likely an even higher proportion for hospitals in the small towns.[64] We know that payments into the Social Security Trust Fund from rural populations have been lower than from urban, so that this program has probably yielded some redistribution of national wealth toward strengthening rural health care resources.

Medicare has also had another important effect of potentially great importance for rural areas. Since many billions of new dollars were injected into the health services without any significant change in delivery patterns, medical prices rose steeply. Demands for care continued to mount, and people of all social classes, especially the poor, found service increasingly difficult to get. In July 1969 the White House was led to issue a statement saying:

This nation is faced with a breakdown in the delivery of health care unless immediate concerted action is taken by the government and the private sector. Expansion of private and public financing has created a demand for services far in excess of the capacity of our health system to respond.

With widespread talk of a "national crisis in health care," a whole series of new legislative proposals were made to extend the social insurance principle to the whole national population. These proposals varied from government subsidy of membership for low-income people in voluntary health insurance plans to mandatory enrollment of all working people in existing plans to universal coverage of the entire national population.[65] Most remarkable is the fact that a Republican national administration, long opposed to any compulsion in health insurance enrollment, in 1973 advocated compulsory payment of health insurance premiums by all employers in the nation—albeit with various deductibles and cost-sharing features for the patient. Also remarkable is the advocacy of legislative incentives to modify traditional delivery patterns, that is, private solo practice and fee-for-service remuneration, by both major political parties.

All of the recently proposed national health insurance bills would bring some new benefits for rural people, but the greatest would undoubtedly come from legislation that would achieve a centralized flow of social insurance funds. These could then be reallocated to local geographic areas in some reasonable relationship to the health needs of each community. Only a program on the classical model of our present social security system (like the "Health Security Bill" of 1972) would do this. As of this writing, the outcome of these debates is quite uncertain, and it will obviously depend on larger political events. One can be quite certain, however, that some new legislation will soon be enacted to provide stronger economic support for general medical care, and that such action will have particular value for rural populations.

Health planning

Most of the movements for improvement in rural health service that we have reviewed imply a type of social planning. When the American Medical Association set out to "grade" medical schools after the Flexner Report of 1910, that constituted health manpower planning. When Titles V and VI of the Social Security Act of 1935 called for state plans in maternal and child health and general public health, as a condition for federal grants, that was health service planning. The state "master plans" for hospital construction under the Hill-Burton Act of 1946 compelled facility planning even more obviously. During World War II there was extensive activity on "postwar planning," including commissions in every state, stimulated by the Agricultural Extension Service, for rural health service improvements.[66]

However, in 1966, soon after Medicare, the first federal legislation specifically in support of "comprehensive health planning" was enacted at the state and local (or "areawide") levels.[67] This was largely stimulated by the multiplicity of federal grant-in-aid programs for categorical health purposes that had accumulated over the years, each requiring its own special administrative review. The new law consolidated most (though not all) of these into one block health grant to a single health agency, at which point decisions would be made on allocations of the money for different purposes. To make these decisions, there were to be set up state "Comprehensive Health Planning Councils" of which consumers must constitute a majority. Corresponding CHP boards were also financed in local areas, into which each state had to be divided, but the functions of these local boards have not been so explicit. New funds were also made available for "innovative" health service programs in local communities (Public Health Service Act Section 314-e), not within the scope of the "formula grant" for overall purposes received by each state.[68]

The CHP legislation calls for planning of "health manpower, facilities, and services"—a broad enough scope, but without much mandatory authority, except as it has been or will be established by subsequent legislation. The most active role of CHP boards has probably been with regard to planning the construction of facilities, and the staffing of many of these boards has been derived from the earlier councils devoted exclusively to hospital planning. Some twenty states have now passed legislation requiring "certificates of need," approved by a CHP agency, for any new hospital construction, regardless of whether governmental subsidy is received or not.[69]

The CHP movement has special meaning for rural areas because the free market determination of the allocation of resources, especially in health manpower, has obviously not been adequately responsive to human needs. Only where market mechanisms have been modified, as in the Hill-Burton, the OEO, or the Medicare-Medicaid programs, have rural areas seen solid health care improvements. At some future time, when overall funds for health service are more systematically allocated, one may expect that the CHP movement will acquire real force. In the meantime, many consumers of health care are getting educated about the problems. In 1974 the National Health Planning and Resources Development Act (P.L. 93-641) marked an important new stage in this developmental process.

A major impetus to health planning in recent years, aside from the earmarked legislative support, has obviously been the rising costs of medical care. This has been going on, of course, for many decades, but until about 1950 the rise in our gross national productivity (GNP) and national income went along at a corresponding pace, so that health costs remained at between 3.5% and 4.5% of our GNP.[70] Since 1950, health costs have been rising at a noticeably greater rate than the GNP, and today they exceed 8%. This has resulted from rises both in rates of utilization and in prices per unit of service. It is these cost pressures that have largely stimulated so much of the concern for training new types of allied health personnel, noted earlier, and for achieving greater efficiency in the operation of hospitals, which remains the most expensive component of health care.[71]

Another important outcome of the cost pressures, with special meaning for rural populations, has been the new official national promotion of "health maintenance organizations" (HMO's). In a "Health Strategy" message of February 1971, President Nixon called for nationwide promotion of HMO's as one of the soundest approaches to cost-containment along with quality controls.[72] The idea of providing persons with a relatively comprehensive range of physician, hospital, and related services for a fixed annual premium is, of course, not new; what is new is its promotion by government. Patterns of delivery of service under HMO's may still involve private solo medical practice and fee payments by "medical foundations," although the commonest interpretation has assumed the more organized framework of group practice clinics, where systematic preventive and curative services, as well as quality assurance, can be better arranged. There are various hazards of underservicing in the HMO concept, which, most observers agree, will require careful governmental surveillance if the pattern becomes widespread through public financial support. After extended debate, the Health Maintenance Organization Act (P.L. 93-222) was enacted by Congress in December 1973; it authorized $375 million over a 5-year period for promoting and assisting establishment of new HMO's, with special priorities for covering populations in underserviced rural areas.

For rural populations the HMO pattern could have the special advantage of mobilizing many different types of health resource in isolated areas. Patients would not have to wend their way through a dispersed pluralistic maze to get integrated health care. In a sense, the HMO idea, if backed up by adequate financial support, would constitute a characteristically American approach to the planning of total health services, the initiative coming from many local communities instead of being mandated by a central power. Opportunities for strong consumer input, furthermore, into the methods by which health needs are met would be greater than ever before.

Conclusions

In conclusion, I shall not try to summarize these several streams of increasing organization of rural health services in America. I will just offer a few general observations on what seem to me to be the prominent overall trends.

From early attention focused on disease prevention, the movement has widened to social concern for comprehensive health service. While the preventive focus was understandably warranted in a period of dramatic new discoveries in community hygiene, the technical inseparability of prevention and treatment and the greater social effectiveness of their combination has become increasingly appreciated.

The interdependence of actions in the several sectors of health service has become increasingly recognized as necessary for rural improvements. Programs for facility construction, manpower expansion, economic support, and quality promotion are all obviously intertwined. These actions, in turn, are all interdependent with general social changes in agriculture, employment, transportation, education, social security, and other spheres. Reaching goals in any one of these sectors usually depends on parallel actions in several of the others.

Health service improvements, it has become clear, cannot be left to the initiative of physicians and other health professionals alone. Progress has come largely from the demands of consumers, expressing their will through various citizen organizations and ultimately through elected representatives in government. In fact, much of the progress has been achieved over the opposition of leaders of the private medical profession. This does not mean that consumers could work effectively without sound technical advice, but such advice has been available from many sources.

Because of the complexities and rising costs of health service, improvement has become increasingly dependent on collective economic efforts. The mechanisms of private spending or of charity have become gradually replaced by insurance or tax support. Along with this, people have naturally become more and more concerned with how wisely the collectively raised monies are spent for health service.

As public knowledge of the health sciences has widened, professional discipline has heightened and greater social controls over the quality of services have been developed. These have emanated from both governmental and private sources, but all of them have meant greater social organization of resources.

Significant rural health improvements, it has become quite clear, cannot be expected within the boundaries of rural communities themselves. Cooperation is needed from the cities, along both economic and technical lines.

As the instrumentality for linking rural and urban resources, government has had to play an increasing role. This means government at all levels, but the main thrust has come from state and national, rather than town and county levels. National and state taxing powers have been the major vehicles for redistribution of resources, to achieve greater equity for rural people.

At present, marked deficiencies still characterize rural health service, compared with the potential levels that have been shown to be attainable in the cities. This is seen in affluent America as much as or more than it is seen in many other countries of lesser wealth. The main lesson of history would seem to be that future reduction of rural deficiencies in health resources and services will depend largely on deliberate social actions by the national government.

References

1. Hall, W. W.: Health of farmers' families. In Report: commissioner of agriculture for 1862, Washington, D.C., 1862, U.S. Government Printing Office, p. 453.

2. Hall, W. W.: Farmers' homes. In Report: commissioner of agriculture for 1863, Washington, D.C., 1863, U.S. Government Printing Office, pp. 313 ff.

3. Roemer, M. I.: Historic development of the

current crisis of rural medicine in the United States. In Victor Robinson memorial volume: essays on historical medicine, New York, 1948, Froben Press, pp. 333-342.

4. Shattuck, L.: Report of the Sanitary Commission of Massachusetts 1850, reprinted, Cambridge, 1948, Harvard University Press.

5. Mustard, H. S.: Rural health practice, New York, 1936, Commonwealth Fund, pp. 4 ff.

6. The Rockefeller Foundation: Annual report, 1940, The Rockefeller Foundation.

7. Roemer, M. I., and Faulkner, B.: The development of public health services in a rural county: 1838-1949, J. Hist. Med. 1: 22-43, 1951.

8. Lumsden, L. L.: Extent of rural health service in the U.S. 1926-30, Public Health Rep. 45: 1065-1081, May 9, 1930.

9. Mustard, H. S.: Government in public health, New York, 1945, Commonwealth Fund, pp. 73-77.

10. Vaughan, H. F.: Local health services in the United States: the story of the CAP, Am. J. Public Health 62:95-111, January 1972.

11. Schottland, C. I.: The social security program in the United States, New York, 1963, Appleton-Century-Crofts.

12. Kratz, F. W.: Status of full-time local health organizations at the end of fiscal year 1941-42, Public Health Rep. 58:345-351, February 26, 1943.

13. Emerson, H.: Local health units for the nation, New York, 1945, Commonwealth Fund.

14. U.S. Public Health Service: Directory of local health units 1964, PHS Pub. No. 118, revised, Washington, D.C., 1964, U.S. Government Printing Office.

15. Roemer, M. I.: Health needs and services of the rural poor. In Rural poverty in the United States, Washington, D.C., 1968, National Commission on Rural Poverty, pp. 311-332.

16. Rosen, G.: Fees and fee bills: some economic aspects of medical practice in 19th century America, Bull. Hist. Med. (Suppl.) 6:16-18, 1946.

17. Moore, H. H.: American medicine and the people's health, New York, 1927, The Macmillan Co., p. 195.

18. Roemer, M. I.: Approaches to the rural doctor shortage, Rural Sociology 16:137-147, June 1951.

19. Shanholtz, M. I.: Virginia State Department of Health, personal communication, April 3, 1967.

20. Massie, W. A.: Medical services for rural areas: the Tennessee Medical Foundation, Cambridge, 1957, Harvard University Press.

21. M.D.'s obtained for rural areas, AMA News, February 27, 1967.

22. Madison, D. L.: A rural health care strategy for the Robert Wood Johnson Foundation, Chapel Hill, September 1972 (processed), University of North Carolina, Rural Health Services Research Unit.

23. Coggeshall, L. T.: Planning for medical progress through education, Evanston, Ill., 1965, Association of American Medical Colleges.

24. Report of the National Advisory Commission on Health Manpower, vol. I, Washington, D.C., 1967, U.S. Government Printing Office.

25. U.S. Department of Health, Education and Welfare: Inventory of federal programs that support health manpower training, Washington, D.C., November 1971, U.S. Government Printing Office.

26. Field, M. G.: Soviet socialized medicine, New York, 1967, The Free Press.

27. Health personnel will be assigned to critical manpower-lacking areas, Med. Tribune, June 28, 1972.

28. Southmayd, H. J., and Smith, G.: Small community hospitals, New York, 1944, Commonwealth Fund.

29. Mott, F. D., and Roemer, M. I.: Rural health and medical care, New York, 1948, McGraw-Hill Book Co., pp. 384-386.

30. Mountin, J. W., Pennell, E. H., and Hoge, V. M.: Health service areas—requirements for general hospitals and health centers, Public Health Service, Bulletin No. 292, Washington, D.C., 1945, U.S. Government Printing Office.

31. Commission on Hospital Care: Hospital care in the United States, Chicago, 1946, Commission on Hospital Care.

32. U.S. Public Health Service: Two decades of partnership: Hill-Burton Program 1946-1966, PHS Pub. No. 930-F-9, Washington, D.C., August 1966, U.S. Government Printing Office.

33. Roemer, M. I.: The distribution of hospital beds needed in a region, J. Health Hum. Behav. 1:94-101, Summer 1960.

34. U.S. Department of Health, Education and

Welfare: To improve medical care—a guide to federal financial aid for the development of medical care services, facilities, personnel, Washington, D.C., April 1966, U.S. Government Printing Office, p. 49.

35. Mott, F. D., and Roemer, M. I.: *op. cit.,* pp. 389-431.

36. Mott, F. D., and Roemer, M. I.: A federal program of public health and medical services for migratory farm workers, Public Health Rep. 60:229-249, March 2, 1945.

37. U.S. Senate, Committee on Labor and Public Welfare: The migratory farm labor problem in the United States, 1965, Report No. 155, Washington, D.C., 1965, U.S. Government Printing Office.

38. U.S. Public Health Service: Health services for American Indians, PHS Pub. No. 531, Washington, D.C., 1957, U.S. Government Printing Office.

39. Wagner, C. J., and Rabeau, E. S.: Indian poverty and Indian health, HEW Indicators, March 1964, pp. 24-44.

40. Schorr, L. B., and English, J. T.: Background, context and significant issues in neighborhood health center programs, Milbank Mem. Fund Q. 46:289-296, July 1968.

41. Elinson, J., and Herr, C. E. A.: A sociomedical view of neighborhood health centers, Med. Care 8:97-103, March-April 1970.

42. Williams, P.: The purchase of medical care through fixed periodic payment, New York, 1932, National Bureau of Economic Research.

43. United Mine Workers of America Welfare and Retirement Fund: Report for the year ending June 30, 1972, Washington, D.C., 1972.

44. Munts, R.: Bargaining for health: labor unions, health insurance and medical care, Madison, Wis., 1967, University of Wisconsin Press, p. 141.

45. Rosenfeld, L. S., and Makover, H. B.: The Rochester Regional Hospital Council, Cambridge, 1956, Harvard University Press.

46. McNerney, W. J., and Riedel, D. C.: Regionalization and rural health care, Ann Arbor, 1962, University of Michigan Bureau of Hospital Administration.

47. de la Chapelle, C. E., and Jensen, F.: A mission in action—the story of the Regional Hospital Plan of New York University, New York, 1964, New York University Press.

48. Marston, R. Q.: A nation starts a program: regional medical programs 1965-66, J. Med. Educ., January 1967, pp. 17-27.

49. Bodenheimer, T. S.: Regional medical programs: no road to regionalization, Med. Care Rev. 26:1125-1166, December 1969.

50. Ross, A., and Boyle, R. L., Jr.: Urban-rural exchange programs, Hospitals, July 16, 1972, pp. 55-59.

51. U.S. Public Health Service: Medical groups in the United States, PHS Pub. No. 1063, Washington, D.C., July 1963, U.S. Government Printing Office.

52. Jordan, E. P.: The physician in group practice, Chicago, 1958, Year Book Medical Publishers, Inc.

53. Somers, A. R.: Hospital regulation: the dilemma of public policy, Princeton, N.J., 1969, Princeton University, Industrial Relations Section.

54. Roemer, M. I.: Health needs and services of the rural poor, *op. cit.*

55. Goldmann, F.: Public medical care: principles and problems, New York, 1945, Columbia University Press.

56. Myers, R. J.: Medicare, Homewood, Ill., 1970, Richard D. Erwin.

57. U.S. Senate, Committee on Finance: Medicare and Medicaid: problems, issues, and alternatives, Washington, D.C., February 9, 1970, U.S. Government Printing Office.

58. Somers, H. M., and Somers, A. R.: Doctors, patients, and health insurance, Washington, D.C., 1961, The Brookings Institution.

59. U.S. National Center for Health Statistics: Health insurance coverage, United States 1962-63, PHS Pub. No. 1000, Series 10, No. 11, Washington, D.C., 1964, U.S. Government Printing Office.

60. Reed, L. S.: The extent of health insurance coverage in the United States, Washington, D.C., 1964, U.S. Social Security Administration, Research Report No. 10.

61. Shadid, M. A.: Doctors of today and tomorrow, New York, 1947, Cooperative League of America.

62. Harris, R.: A sacred trust, New York, 1966, The New American Library, Inc.

63. Feingold, E.: Medicare: policies and politics, San Francisco, 1966, Chandler Publishing Co.

64. U.S. Social Security Administration: The impact of Medicare: an annotated bibliography of selected sources, Washington, D.C., 1969, U.S. Government Printing Office.

65. Falk, I. S.: National health insurance: a review of policies and proposals, Law Contemp. Probl. **35:**669-696, Autumn 1970.

66. U.S. Department of Agriculture, Inter-Bureau Committee on Post-War Programs: Better health for rural America, Washington, D.C., October 1945, U.S. Government Printing Office.

67. Stewart, W. H.: New dimensions of health planning, Chicago, 1967, University of Chicago, Graduate School of Business Administration.

68. Cater, D., Willard, W. R., Sax, E. D., and Rogers, P. G.: Comprehensive health planning, Am. J. Public Health **58:**1022-1038, 1968.

69. Anderson, N. N.: Comprehensive health planning in the states: a study and critical analysis, Minneapolis, Minn., December 1968, American Rehabilitation Foundation.

70. Rice, D. P., and Cooper, B. S.: National health expenditures 1929-70, Soc. Security Bull., January 1971, pp. 3-18.

71. National Advisory Commission on Health Facilities: A report to the President, Washington, D.C., December 1968, U.S. Government Printing Office.

72. Klarman, H. E.: Analysis of the HMO proposal—its assumptions, implications, and prospects. In Health maintenance organizations: a reconfiguration of the health services system, Chicago, 1971, University of Chicago Center for Health Administration Studies, pp. 24-38.

CHAPTER 2 Development of public health services in a rural county

Governmental public health activities started in the larger cities, where environmental sanitation and communicable disease control presented special problems. In small towns, and particularly the rural districts around them, such official services were slow to develop; in the nineteenth century the actions taken were largely regulatory and punitive.

By tracing developments in one predominantly rural county over the last century, the evolution of the public health movement in America can be seen, from its originally narrow scope and local base of authority to its present wider scope and national base of authority and support. One can discern the widening concern for personal health services, as distinguished from purely environmental controls. Parallel with this are the several administrative changes in the structure of public health agencies and the relationships of local to state and federal authorities. In the 25 years since this paper was written, the scope of public health services has obviously broadened further, and the administrative relationships have become more complex.

The research for tracing this history was done while the author served as Health Officer of Monongalia County, West Virginia in 1948-1949. With the coauthorship of Barbara Faulkner, this paper was published as "The Development of Public Health Services in a Rural County: 1838-1949" in *Journal of the History of Medicine and Allied Sciences* **1**:22-43, January 1951.

In the day-to-day public health service of a community, much of which is quiet vigilance, devoid of the drama of the hospital or clinic, it is easy to lose sight of the great progress made over the last century. In back of some of the most elementary features of the modern health program lies a long story of exploration, controversy, and slow technical development. The approval of a septic tank installation, the immunization of a child, the x-ray examination of an adult's chest may be taken for granted today, but the full significance of these measures can be appreciated only by tracing their historical development.

The history of the acquisition of the knowledge on which public health activities are based goes back to antiquity and traces its roots to all parts of the civilized world. The story of the application of this knowledge on a community basis, however—of public health organization—can be found in the records of many communities. In fact, an account of the evolution of organized health services in almost any locality in the United States reflects the developments of public health throughout the nation. Such a study has been made in Monongalia County, West Virginia.

Monongalia County is in the north central part of West Virginia, on the southern border of Pennsylvania, better known as the Mason-Dixon line. It has a population of about 60,000, and its principal town, Morgantown, is the site of West Virginia University. While the county is rural by the usual Census Bureau definition (over 65% of its people live in places of under 2500 population), only about 10% of the residents are engaged in farming. The largest single occupational group consists of miners, who, with their families, make up about one-third of the county population. There are a number of small industries in the county and a relatively large white-collar class associated with the University.

As rural counties go, Monongalia County has an active public health program, with a County Health Department housed in a modern health center, staffed by a full-time health officer, public health nurses, sanitarians, clerks, and other technical personnel. Its program includes activities in environmental sanitation, acute and chronic communicable disease control, maternal and child health services, vital statistics, laboratory services, health education, dental hygiene, cancer control, and many other aspects of community health service. By current optimal standards there are many inadequacies, but some appreciation of what has been accomplished so far in this and hundreds of other communities may be gleaned by looking backward a century or more.

Early efforts in sanitary control and medical care for the poor (1838-1890)

The year 1911 has become so firmly established in the public health literature as the date of the first full-time health department in a rural county that one may easily overlook how much that is germane to rural public health was done long before this. Official community concern for the systematic prevention of disease in Monongalia County is found at least as early as 1838. In that year the Common Council of the City of Morgantown, which was at this time still part of Virginia, enacted an ordinance forbidding the disposal of rubbish or trash in the streets of the city. Anyone doing so was liable to fine and payment of the cost of the removal of the refuse.*

The general relationship between filth and disease had long been recognized,[12] and numerous steps were taken to reduce the accumulation of dirt. In 1849 the Morgantown City Council ordained that no person be allowed to build a hogpen in any street or alley of the city. Two years later it was decreed that any sow or hog found running loose on city streets would be captured and sold, the city retaining the sales price as a fine. Undoubtedly, aesthetic considerations figured prominently in legal prohibitions of this type. Yet this was the period of general sanitary awakening, almost of the very year of Shattuck's *Report of the Sanitary Commission of Massachusetts* (1850), and hygienic motivations doubtless were equally important.

Almost as early as concern for a sanitary environment in Morgantown was

---

*For the primary sources on which the main body of this paper is based, see references 1-11.

official action in the sphere of medical care for the indigent. In the absence of any official supervisor of the poor, the City Council voted that two dollars be paid to Miss Hatfield for attending Mrs. Shroyer during her illness and that Mr. George Chalfant be allowed five dollars for nursing John Achinson during his illness. Similar payments are recorded in 1854. It is significant perhaps that payments to physicians are not indicated, but that, in the absence of a hospital in the county, nursing care of a sort was provided.

In March 1855 the first official action was taken to control a specific communicable disease. The General Assembly of Virginia had passed a law granting municipalities the power to prevent injury or annoyance to any citizen from anything "dangerous, unhealthy, or offensive." Under this authorization, the borough required that the head of each household see that every member of the house was vaccinated against smallpox. All physicians or other persons, moreover, visiting a home afflicted with smallpox were required to use proper precautions and disinfecting measures to protect other citizens. A Virginia statute in 1861 required appointment of a state official to furnish material for vaccination.[13]

Virginia amended its charter to Morgantown in 1860, incorporating in it specific power for the City Council to take action "to prevent injury and annoyance to the public from anything dangerous, offensive or unwholesome." A number of additional sanitary ordinances were promptly enacted. It was proclaimed unlawful to deposit any nuisance or dead animal in the town limits. Doubtless inspired by miasmatic conceptions, it became unlawful for any person to have stagnant water on his or her property. Any owner or occupant of property with an accumulation of garbage or filth offensive or injurious to health had to have it removed immediately. Excreta disposal entered official purview with a law requiring that any person owning a privy within the town limits that was a nuisance or injurious to health must have it removed or keep it in proper order. Doubtless to reduce odors and insects, slaughtering of animals in the city limits was forbidden from April 1 to November 1.

Whether or not there was any effective enforcement of these sanitary prohibitions is difficult to say. If this small town was like the great cities of the day, however, the likelihood of enforcement was small.[14] Even in the larger cities of the period, the rudimentary boards of health rarely convened except in epidemic situations, doing little or nothing on a day-to-day basis. As it happens, it is claimed that two of the earliest boards of health in the nation had been established in Morgantown's mother state at the time, in Petersburg and Alexandria, Virginia, in 1780 and 1804, respectively,[15] but there is little evidence that they functioned. No sign of a permanent or even transient board of health is found for Monongalia County until some years later.

It is likely that the general disruption caused by the Civil War delayed the organization of civic government for health purposes in Monongalia

County. Morgantown was one of the centers of antislavery feeling in the Old Dominion of Virginia. This was the very battleground of the war between the states, the first land battle of the war being fought at Phillippi, only about forty miles to the south. In the midst of the war the mountainous western portion of Virginia, which was not tied to the South by a plantation economy, broke off from the Old Dominion, forming in 1863 the state of West Virginia. It was not until 1869, 4 years after the end of hostilities, that the first state board of health in the nation was organized in Massachusetts; West Virginia did not establish such a board until 1881.[16] Ten years later, in 1891, the state of West Virginia authorized the county courts to establish county boards of health.

Boards of health in county and city (1891-1918)

Apparently little time was then lost, and in the same year, 1891, the Monongalia County Court appointed its first Board of Health. The composition of the first board is not clear, but 3 years later it consisted of a physician and two laymen appointed by the court and directed to work in cooperation with the president of the County Court and the county prosecuting attorney. The first reference to enforcement of sanitary ordinances is found in 1891 when the City Council of Morgantown requested the new County Board of Health to investigate all points in the town about which complaints had been made or that they considered objectionable and to report in writing places needing regulation by the City Council. Two years later, on July 17, 1893, such a report was made. The City Council voted to visit personally the places indicated. They did this the next day and ordered these places to be cleaned.

Further progress was made in the provision of medical care for the indigent in 1892. In that year the County Court appointed a physician on a salary of $300 a year to provide care for the poor of Morgantown and the area immediately around the city. A separate physician was appointed by the City Council in 1897-1898 at a part-time salary of $65 a year to provide care for the sick poor of Morgantown. The town physician's salary had fallen to $40 a year in 1900, but by 1903 it had risen to $150.

The first extension of sanitary regulations since the antebellum period is found in 1895 when the Morgantown City Council passed an ordinance on public sewers. A street commissioner, whose duties were to supervise sewers in all public streets, alleys, and wharves, was appointed. Private sewer lines connecting homes or other establishments with the public sewers had to be kept in proper condition by the property owner.

In 1899 the city of Morgantown created a separate Board of Health consisting not of independent citizens, like the county board, but of the mayor, the recorder, and the town physician (for the sick poor). Perhaps because its functions were being performed by the county board, or perhaps for other reasons, in 1902 the city board was abolished.

It appears likely that the executive authorities of the County Board of Health were actually exercised by its physician member. On April 21, 1903 the *Morgantown Post* reported the resignation of Mr. E. McL. Warren from the board of health, referring to him as the "county health officer," because he was dissatisfied with the low remuneration for his work. The next month another physician was appointed in his place, designated in the County Court *Miscellaneous Order Book* as "health officer." He received $600 in this capacity, plus $3 for every day a communicable disease case was under quarantine, a sum that might be very large, indeed, if actually paid. The part-time county health officer, still found in hundreds of rural counties, had entered the scene.

The very same year, in December 1903, the city of Morgantown took parallel action, appointing its first city health officer at a salary of $75 a month. Since the new county health officer was responsible for the entire county (with the city in it), there was clearly a jurisdictional problem and a special meeting was held between the mayor of Morgantown and the County Court to work it out. It was decided that the city health officer would serve as the agent of the County Court within the borders of Morgantown and the county health officer would be responsible for the rest of the county. The duties of the city health officer were stated to include visiting cases of communicable disease, quarantining houses when necessary, inspecting sewers, fumigating houses, and keeping account of contagious diseases occurring in town.

Morgantown continued to develop new methods of providing care for the needy. In 1900 the first hospital was established in the county. As in so many rural sections, it was launched by a group of physicians as a private venture, unlike the first urban hospitals, which had been started 150 years earlier as public or charitable institutions. In 1903, instead of appointing one city physician for the poor, the City Council made a contract with the new hospital. The task must have been beset with problems, for the next year the arrangement was again changed and two independent physicians were appointed to serve the sick poor. The following year, the city reverted again to the appointment of a single physician for the poor.

Toward the turn of the century, in the boisterous expansion of free enterprise, America had become flooded with patent medicines. The newspapers were filled with advertisements of magic potions that would cure everything from rheumatism to consumption. At the same time, thoughtful men were beginning to expose the treachery of cure-alls and pressing for legislation to curb the false claims of the proprietary drug manufacturers. Finally, in the trust-busting administration of Theodore Roosevelt, under the technical leadership of Dr. Harvey Wiley of the United States Department of Agriculture, the first Pure Food and Drug law was passed by Congress in 1906.[17] This federal law applied only to nostrums sold in interstate commerce; similar action had been proposed or passed within the states since the 1880's. Against this background it is significant that in 1905 the Morgantown City Council enacted an ordinance making it unlawful for anyone to sell diseased, corrupted, unwholesome, impure, or adulterated food or drink within the city. It was also deemed unlawful for anyone to misrepresent any product (presumably including drugs) sold in the city.

From 1903 on, both the county and the city had part-time health officers, although there was a large turnover in these positions. The first sign of relative stability was seen in 1909, when Dr. Charles H. McLane was appointed by the court as county health officer for a 4-year term, and reappointed for another 4-year term in 1913. In this period the county health officer began to give quarterly reports on contagious diseases to the County Court.

Meanwhile, in 1907 the city of Morgantown reestablished its separate Board of Health, which had been abandoned in 1902. It was broadened now to consist of two citizens, as well as the mayor, the city attorney, and a physician. The medical member was now not the physician for the poor, however, but the city health officer. The city board had the same powers as were authorized by the 1891 West Virginia State Statute for the county board. It was to report any insanitary conditions to the mayor for correction and was empowered to make rules deemed necessary to protect the health of the city. This delegation of law-making responsibilities by the council to the Board of Health was something new and quite significant. The first rules, adopted in 1908, concerned the sanitary maintenance of stables in the city, the removal of manure, and the control of garbage and refuse disposal. Quite important was a regulation that where public sewers were accessible, all outside privies be eliminated. The city health officer was empowered to enforce communicable disease quarantines.

The first publicly organized system of garbage disposal in the county was begun in Morgantown in 1907. In May of that year the City Council appointed a garbage committee, which took a 30-day option on some lots. A man was to be employed to burn any garbage hauled to this dumping area. Six years later, in 1913, action was taken to appoint a superintendent of the city incinerating plant. It was ordained further that all garbage in the city or in transit was to be kept in watertight metallic containers.

While the lines of development of the city and county public health program, on one hand, and the city and county system for medical care of the poor, on the other, were all legally distinct, a review of the actual personalities involved suggests much overlapping. One physician was the county's physician for the poor one year and the city health officer the next; another was city health officer and one of the city's physicians for the poor at the same time. There were manifestly jurisdictional delineations between the civic officials of city and county governments, but the appointments of both political units had to be made from the same small group of physicians. The sharp lines now usually seen between public health administration and medical care programs for the indigent were still rather fuzzy.

As the city of Morgantown grew, there came to the fore another major health problem incident especially to urban life—the safety of milk. As long as scattered farms each distributed milk to only a handful of families, the problem was not striking, but when large numbers of families in a city were reached by a single dairy, the hazard of epidemics loomed. Even a metropolis like New York City did not undertake systematic dairy inspection until 1906, however[18]; Morgantown directed attention to the problem in 1908. The City Council resolved that the sanitary officer must visit any dairy selling milk products within the city to determine if the milk was being handled in a sanitary manner. Any infectious disease in the dairyman's family or the helpers was to be reported to the City Board of Health by the sanitary officer, and he was to check the health of the herds, including tuberculin testing of the cows.

It will be noted that this action refers to a "sanitary officer," but there is no evidence that such a person was appointed, apart from the part-time physician serving as health officer. Further steps in milk sanitation were taken in 1913 when an ordinance was passed that no person could sell in the city any milk that was unclean, came from diseased animals, or had been handled in an unclean manner or milk that was of substandard quality, adulterated, or misrepresented in any way. Dairies were to be inspected four times a year and graded according to scorecards of the Bureau of Animal Husbandry of the United States Department of Agriculture. A city milk inspector was to be appointed by the council to enforce this law and to issue permits to all qualified dealers. The city health officer was to examine all milk handlers and to exclude any with contagious diseases. In 1915 the *City Council Journal* finally recorded the actual appointment of a milk inspector, Mr. J. L. Case, at a salary of $25 per month plus expenses. If this official was a full-time inspector, which is not certain, he may be regarded as the first regular staff member of a public health agency in the county. It may not be unrelated that in 1913 the West Virginia legislature appropriated funds for its first full-time state health officer and established its state hygienic laboratory.

In the slow evolution of democratic institutions, the year 1914 may have a place in Monongalia County history. With the suffrage movement reaching a crescendo that was to lead 6 years later to the Nineteenth Amendment, Mrs. J. P. Fitch became the first woman to be appointed to the City Board of Health.

The health problems related to mobilization of men in the First World War were bound to have an impact on Monongalia County. Among the most important of these was venereal disease, a problem whose extent was shockingly impressed on the nation by the findings of the first million draft examinations.[19] The first national Venereal Disease Act was passed by Congress in July 1918, and in April 1919 the Morgantown City Council took local action. Syphilis, gonorrhea, and chancroid were declared by the council to be contagious diseases that must be reported to the City Board of Health by physicians or hospital superintendents. These reports were to be kept confidential. The city health officer was required to protect others from venereal infection by quarantining persons if necessary. He was also authorized to examine anyone suspected of having venereal disease. In the same ordinance, the local police were called on to prevent the spread of venereal disease through prostitution, and the very spreading of it was declared unlawful.

Growth of personal health services (1919-1928)

Until 1919 all official health activity in the county had related to environmental sanitation, communicable disease control, and medical care of the indigent. In 1919 a new concept appeared—the positive promotion of health through attention to the child. Under the stimulus of the labor movement, the Children's Bureau had been set up in the United States Department of Labor in 1912 to investigate and report on matters pertaining to the welfare of children.[20] From this time a movement was under way to provide federal funds for grants to the states to support organized child health services, resulting finally in the Sheppard-Towner Act for the Promotion of the Welfare of Maternity and Infancy in 1921. Throughout the nation, women, who were taking an increasing part in public life, were promoting measures to protect the development of the child.

In this spirit a group of Morgantown women launched Baby Week in May 1919. An infant clinic was held at which local physicians and nurses donated their services. A representative of the Children's Bureau of the United States Department of Labor was in town for 3 days lecturing on child care. It was decided to continue with a permanent program, and in July 1919 under the sponsorship of the local chapter of the American Red Cross, an infant welfare station with monthly meetings was opened at the local high school. The Red Cross nurse visited homes to teach mothers about child care. Starting in this way under voluntary agency auspices, it was many years before maternal and child health services became a fixed part of the official public health program.

The following year a further step was taken in the interests of child health when the Morgantown Board of Education appointed Miss Genevieve Smith as a full-time school nurse. This was the first appointment of a nurse by an official agency for public health purposes. A year later, in July 1921, Miss Marguerite Clancy was appointed as the first public health nurse to serve the entire county. She worked under the supervision of the part-time county health officer and was paid jointly by the County Court, the Red Cross, and the school boards of the county districts (there were seven separate school districts in the county at the time, not unified under a county board of education until 1935). After only 6 months, however, the County Court stated it could no longer afford to pay its share of the nurse's salary, and the position lapsed.

Under the stimulus of the postwar period and advances in medical knowledge, new developments came in rapid order. In July 1921 child welfare clinics were inaugurated as weekly, instead of monthly, events held in the Morgantown Elks Club. The West Virginia State Department of Health participated now in the management of these clinics, presumably paying physicians and nurses for their services from the new Sheppard-Towner Act funds. This was the first direct health service in the county by the state's official public health agency. A totally new type of clinic, a tuberculosis clinic, was also held in 1921, sponsored by the State Tuberculosis Association, a voluntary agency. Plans were made to hold such clinics monthly in the county courthouse. In August 1922 still another type of clinic, a clinic to treat "social disease," was inaugurated, again with the support of the State Department of Health.

It was obvious that progress in public health organization was being made in Monongalia County through the stimulus of voluntary and official agencies at the state level. But then, as now, local public health organization was believed most stable, and in 1922 the State Health Commissioner, Dr. T. R. Henslow, appealed to the county court to finance a local health department with a full-time health officer. This was the first clear proposal along these lines, but the court did not act.

In 1922 still another segment of health service came under the wing of community action. The Morgantown Board of Education engaged a dental hygienist to examine students' teeth, clean them, and lecture on their proper care. The school nurse was to follow up cases to see that corrective dental care, recommended by the hygienist, was carried out.

The number of public health personnel continued to increase. In May 1923 a full-time nurse was engaged by the County Tuberculosis Association. A share of her salary was paid by the Metropolitan Life Insurance Company, to whose "industrial" policyholders in the county she rendered special services. This pattern of financing visiting nurse services had started in New York City in 1909. The tuberculosis clinic moved from the county courthouse after it came under the sponsorship of the local voluntary agency, and, after a period in commercial quarters, it moved in 1924 to the Labor Temple on invitation of the Central Labor Union of Monongalia County.

Engagement of public health nurses was finally taking hold, and in July 1923 the City Council authorized engagement of the first full-time nurse under the City Board of Health. A report of activities by this nurse and the part-time city health officer for the year 1924 indicated services to 212 cases of communicable disease, including venereal disease, tuberculosis, scarlet fever, diphtheria, whooping cough, typhoid fever, pneumonia, and measles. Investigations had been made on broken sewers and nuisance complaints, and dairy products were examined every 2 or 3 months. A new sanitary service, monthly inspection of restaurants, was reported this year for the first time. The first specific ordinance on restaurant sanitation was not enacted by the city council until 3 years later, in 1927, and this was limited largely to provision that food-handlers be free from contagious disease.

The venereal disease clinic started by the State Health Department in 1922 must have lapsed, for in 1924 the establishment of a permanent service again came under discussion. A cooperative enterprise was planned in which the state would contribute drugs and equipment, the city would provide the services of the city public health nurse and part-time city health officer, the County Tuberculosis Association would lend its nurse, and the county would provide the assistance of its part-time health officer and space in the county courthouse. At the last moment, however, the County Court decided the courthouse should not be used for such a purpose and the whole matter was dropped. These tales of failure are worth recording, for they remind us of the long trail to be blazed before stability is achieved in a service now regarded as elementary as a VD clinic.

Increasingly serious attention was being given to health services for schoolchildren. Systematic examinations by the part-time county health officer, assisted by the Tuberculosis Association nurse and the county home demonstration agent of the Agricultural Extension Service, were begun in rural schools in 1924. A report of the school health program the following year stressed the follow-up to secure the correction of physical defects by nursing visits to the home, the inclusion of health education in the school curriculum, and the physical education program.

It was not until 1926 that a public system of garbage collection was inaugurated in Morgantown. A city disposal area had been maintained since 1907, but haulage of garbage had been private. A superintendent of sanitation was made responsible for the collection and disposal of all refuse, under the direction of the city manager. This major step was taken only after approval by a popular vote.

In 1926, also, a new and unique type of clinic, a "general health clinic," at which anyone was welcome, was held at three rural villages in the county. Whether these clinics were an effort to provide a general physician's care for rural people or something else, we do not hear of them again.

The city of Morgantown completed construction of a new city hall in 1926. The following year the city government had reached the stage of maturity where it felt the need for its first full-time health officer. The position was apparently not attractive to any of the many local physicians who had served as part-time health officials, and the first full-time medical official in Monongalia County, Dr. H. H. Pierce, came from Prince Edward Island, Canada. Dr. Pierce began work in July 1927 and promptly took over the services in the weekly well-baby clinics, formerly attended by private practitioners. He also reorganized and attended weekly venereal disease clinics.

Smallpox had occurred off and on in rural sections of Monongalia County for many years; in 1919, for example, twelve cases had been reported in one week in the village of Lowsville. When several cases occurred in 1928, however, the county's public health organization was better prepared for action, and the County Court ordered that free vaccination against smallpox be given to all children in the county schools and to adults who could not afford vaccination by a private physician.

It seems likely that the smallpox scare had an impact on public feelings about a full-time health department for the entire county, for only a few months later a petition with 1100 signatures was presented to the County Court requesting a full-time unit. The petition was formally submitted by the County Teachers' Association, the county superintendent of schools, and the county agricultural agent; major legwork in circulation of this petition was done by the farm women's clubs and the parent-teacher associations around the county.

Now that public opinion had been aroused, the County Medical Society, through its president, spoke up against the organization of a full-time county health department. It was charged that such an agency would usurp the rights of the medical profession by immunizing children against smallpox, diphtheria, and typhoid fever. A series of newspaper editorials, however, answered this opposition, and public favor for the idea continued to grow. The division of rural sanitation in the State Department of Health assisted the movement by offering to contribute $5000 toward the total proposed budget of $13,000. The total cost on this basis would be 33 cents per capita of the county population and 1.6 cents per $100 of assessed valuation of property in the county.

A full-time county health department (1929-1935)

Finally, on September 11, 1929, the Monongalia County Court ordered the establishment of a full-time county health department. In December the new department got under way with Dr. R. C. Farrier as the first full-time county health officer, assisted by a public health nurse, a sanitation officer, and a clerk. The first quarters occupied were characteristically in the basement of the county courthouse. At the end of its first year of operations, the County Health Department reported the following activities: (1) health education through newspaper articles, bulletins, and lectures; (2) sanitary inspections of water sources, sewage disposal facilities, dairies, and restaurants; (3) physical examination of food-handlers; (4) quarantining and isolation of cases of acute communicable disease; (5) visits to cases of tuberculosis, dispatch of patients to sanatoria, and assistance at the monthly clinics of the County Tuberculosis Association; (6) operation of a weekly venereal disease clinic; (7) tuberculin tests of cows; (8) immunization of schoolchildren against smallpox, diphtheria, and typhoid fever; (9) infant and preschool child clinics held and home visits made by the nurse; (10) schoolchildren examined and referrals made for correction of physical defects; and (11) births, deaths, and communicable disease recorded. Funds to support this work were contributed by the County Court, the State Health Department, and the United States Public Health Service (through its special rural sanitation grants).

Another new service, a crippled children's clinic, was launched under voluntary auspices in 1929. The County Society for Crippled Children undertook this service, utilizing donated services of physicians.

Meanwhile, the Morgantown City Health Department continued to operate. In 1931 the city adopted the standard milk ordinance recommended by the United States Public Health Service. Since most of the dairies supplying milk to the city were located in the outlying sections of the county, however, inspections were to be made by the county department. Milk sanitation was only one instance of interrelationships, if not duplications, between the city and county public health agencies. It was obvious that this separation of functions could not continue for long. In January 1933 the county health officer appeared before the Morgantown City Council and proposed consolidation of the city and county units. A committee was appointed to investigate the matter, and, instead of consolidation, the council decided to abolish the City Health Department 6 months later. Responsibilities for public health services within the city were finally taken over by the county department.

With a countywide public health agency established, under full-time medical direction, progress continued. School health services were expanded; students were offered prizes for being immunized, for being free from physical defects, and for practicing good health habits. In 1934 venereal disease clinics were increased to twice a week, a schedule that has continued to the present time. In the dark depression years of 1933-1935, however, the funds appropriated for the health department declined, and a skeleton staff of a physician, nurse, sanitarian, and clerk kept at their jobs on presumably reduced salaries. In 1935 the board of education, which had engaged its own dental hygienist for the Morgantown schools since 1922, discontinued this service, and in 1936 the school nurse who had worked in Morgantown since 1920 was released.

National and state impacts on the county (1936-1939)

At this time, when the financial situation in the county was dismal, a major development on the national scene brightened the picture for organized public health everywhere. In 1935 one of the great social measures of our time was launched with the enactment of the Social Security Act. Many had advocated inclusion of social insurance for medical care costs, along with old-age and unemployment protection, but medical opposition was encountered. To facilitate quick passage of this act in an emergency situation, Titles V and VI, which provided federal grants to the states for public health and maternal and child health services, were accepted as a compromise. In 1936 therefore, relatively large sums were granted by the United States Public Health Service and the Children's Bureau to the West Virginia State Department of Health, and some of these funds were passed along to Monongalia County.

These new federal funds enabled the county public health program to keep moving despite the economic depression. In September 1936 the Health

Department was able to add another nurse to its staff, filling the gap left by the termination of the Board of Education's nurse earlier in the year. This marked a beginning of more extensive services by the Health Department within the school system. In this period, also, some financial assistance for the correction of physical defects found in schoolchildren was given by the County Court directly, and by the County Welfare Board. In 1937 a West Virginia state law, which made immunization for both smallpox and diphtheria compulsory for all children entering school, established new responsibilities for the health department in the field of school hygiene.

The rule-making powers granted to the City Board of Health in 1907 were apparently not acted on in the subsequent years. Both City and County Boards of Health gradually became authorities merely on paper. New ordinances were passed by the Morgantown City Council in 1936, bringing various sanitation requirements up to date. Enforcement powers were now clearly given to the county health officer regarding such matters as sewage disposal, garbage collection, and restaurant cleanliness. Restaurants, in fact, were required to have a yearly permit to operate, and such permits could be withheld for sanitary deficiencies.

The countywide scope of the Health Department became more pronounced as well-baby clinics were established in 1937 in three outlying villages. A new type of clinic, a prenatal clinic, was also launched in one of the coal-mining villages. In 1938 still another type of organized service, a weekly "tonsil clinic," was started at which tonsillectomies were to be arranged for children referred by the Health Department and certified by the Department of Public Assistance as being indigent; it was financed by the local Community Chest and public welfare funds.

The entire field of medical care for the indigent had undergone radical changes as a result of other actions by the federal government. In 1933 with the collapse of local relief services everywhere in the nation, the Federal Emergency Relief Administration (FERA) had been set up. This provided federal funds to local communities to pay, among other things, for medical care rendered by any physician to indigent persons. Accordingly, the century-old system of county and city physicians for the poor, paid on part-time annual salaries, was rather abruptly changed in Monongalia County. Nearly all local physicians began to serve indigent persons, submit their bills to the local welfare board, and receive payment on a fee-for-service basis. When the FERA program was replaced by the public assistance provisions of the Social Security Act in 1935, the free choice and fee-for-service system of welfare medicine remained and is still found today.

Still another provision of the Social Security Act influenced Monongalia County in this period. Under Title V, special funds were provided for the rehabilitation of crippled children, and in West Virginia the newly organized State Department of Public Assistance (DPA) was assigned responsibility for administering these funds. A crippled children's clinic rendering limited services had been operating in the county under voluntary auspices since 1929. In 1938 the state DPA set up a monthly clinic for crippled children, attended by an orthopedic surgeon, to serve Monongalia and several surrounding counties. Through this clinic arrangements were made for surgical correction of various orthopedic defects, and it continues to render these services at present. Voluntary agency support for services in the field of child health, however, did not vanish. The Crippled Children's Society continued its work through various forms of supplemental assistance to selected cases. The Morgantown Service League, a women's organization, launched a new well-baby clinic in 1939, paying the nurse and physician with its own funds.

The county's first full-time health officer, Dr. Farrier, remained on the job until September 1936. This seven-year service was the longest of any the county was to have to the present time. The second incumbent remained for about one year, and in October 1937 a change was made that was significant of the whole trend of public health in the nation. On the request of the state government, a commissioned medical officer was assigned to the county by the Federal Public Health Service. He remained as health officer for only 8 months, but this pattern was to be repeated later in 1944 and 1948. The health departments in Monongalia and hundreds of other counties were getting not only money and technical advice from the state and federal governments, but even the loan of trained personnel.

In 1938 Monongalia County was chosen by the West Virgina State Health Department as the field training center for all new public health personnel throughout the state. Public health services everywhere were undergoing rapid expansion; funds were becoming available more rapidly than they could be absorbed for want of competent public health workers. Under the stimulus of federal grants, the state's first field training center had been set up at Beckley in 1935. The location in Morgantown of West Virginia University, founded in 1867, and the general vitality and community support of the Monongalia County program were doubtless reasons for the move. The training center remained a stimulating influence in the County Health Department for over a decade.

In the late 1930's a major campaign to attack venereal disease was launched throughout the nation by the United States Public Health Service. Monongalia County had been directing some attention to this problem since 1919, and VD clinics had been conducted intermittently since 1922, but the federally inspired campaign added new life to local efforts. In October 1938 a local judge spoke out on the menace of syphilis, demanding that houses of prostitution be closed. A few months later, National Social Hygiene Day was observed in the county with the mayor of Morgantown declaring that the city was firmly behind the campaign. The state passed a law in 1939 requiring premarital medical examinations for the detection of syphilis.

Another state law enacted in 1939 reflected the increasing role of state government in local public health affairs. A comprehensive sanitary measure was passed requiring that all systems of water supply, sewage disposal, and garbage disposal meet the approval of the State Department of Health. Statewide legislation of this type takes precedence over all local ordinances passed on the same subjects, except where the local statute is more exacting in its requirements. Between the letter of such laws and their enforcement, however, there was and is a great gap. In 1939 it was reported, for example, that 4500 deficient outdoor privies were located in Monongalia County, although 6413 sanitary privies had been built in the county, mostly by the Work Projects Administration during the previous 5 years.

State government played an increasing role not only legislatively, but also in rendering certain health services directly. Since 1920 local tuberculosis patients had been given hospital care within the county at the small Eastmont Sanatorium. In 1939 the County Court decided it had no further funds with which to support this institution, and it was closed. Henceforth, all local patients with tuberculosis were sent for care to one of three state sanatoria. The facilities of these large state institutions were undoubtedly more adequate.

The current public health program (1940-1949)

By 1940 the County Health Department had become a firm component in community life. Every few years over the previous decade it had moved its quarters to gain more space, and a branch office was now opened in outlying Blackville. In October 1940 the County Health Department was host to the West Virginia State Public Health Conference. In 1942 when Dr. L. A. Mac-Lean, then health officer, was transferred to another county at the behest of the State Department of Health, vigorous protests were issued by several local social agencies and the newspapers.

With the dawn of the Second World War, new forces came into play that resulted in expansion of local public health services. Before Pearl Harbor, industrial mobilization had begun, and a large chemical plant was constructed in Morgantown. Hundreds of new families came to town, and, as in war production centers throughout the country, new problems were created in sanitation, communicable disease control, and other spheres. Restaurant sanitation received new attention; in June 1941 the health officer charged that 98% of Morgantown's restaurants were violating local food ordinances, and another sanitary inspector was engaged to help clean up the situation. The following year, a basic educational approach to the problem of restaurant sanitation was launched, with the initiation of periodic classes of instruction for all food-handlers in the county.

With the lessons of selective service rejections beginning to appear, the County Board of Education decided to do its bit to reduce manpower loss from bad teeth. The dental position, abolished since 1935, was reopened and a hygienist was engaged in 1942 to check the teeth and do prophylaxes on junior and senior high school students.

New technical developments in public health practice found expression in the local program. In 1941 photofluorographic equipment was developed to the point that the State Health Department could send a mobile unit into Monongalia County to take routine chest x-ray films for the detection of tuberculosis. Whooping cough protection was added to the routine immunizations offered in 1942. In 1944 restaurant inspections were put on a firmer technical footing by institution of the bacterial "rim count" technique, with publication of the results in local newspapers.

One of the wartime measures important for public health was the Community Facilities (Lanham) Act, which provided federal funds for construction of hospitals, health centers, and public sanitation facilities in expanded war production areas. Morgantown qualified as such a "defense area," and the County Court applied for the construction of a health center to house the County Health Department. In October 1944 a $39,000 building was completed, adjacent to the Monongalia General Hospital on the edge of Morgantown. The County Health Department had graduated from the courthouse basement of 15 years before to a functional structure with clinical facilities, x-ray and dental equipment, an auditorium, a laboratory, and offices for a well-rounded public health staff.

Two additional organized clinic programs were inaugurated in 1944, in the important fields of cancer and mental disorder. The diagnosis of cancer is a far cry from the traditional service of the public health agency, and it was natural that a cancer diagnostic clinic should be initiated by voluntary agencies. Under the stimulus of the County Field Army of the American Cancer Society, and with the cooperation of the Morgantown Service League and the County Medical Society, a monthly diagnostic clinic was held at the West Virginia University Student Health Center. Later the clinic was transferred to the County Health Center and the Health Department participated actively in its administration. Mental health services were also started with the assistance of the University; they consisted essentially of psychometric examinations of retarded pupils from the county's schools by the department of psychology. The health officer did physical examinations on these youngsters.

In 1945 still another organized service, a dental clinic to do preventive and corrective work on children, was incorporated in the public health program. Referrals to this clinic were made by the dental hygienist working in the schools. With the wartime increase in venereal disease, a new type of worker, a venereal disease field worker, was added to the Health Department staff. This individual worked full time on the epidemiological aspect of venereal disease, aiming to discover all contacts of known cases and bring them under treatment if infected. The County Tuberculosis and Health Association recognized the integral relationship between its program and that of the County Health Department by having its tuberculosis nurse work under the direction of the county health officer.

The Second World War was over in the summer of 1945, and demobilization began. The county health officer, a commissioned officer of the United States Public Health Service who was stationed in the county because of its importance as a war production center, left early in 1946, and the county was without a health officer for 2 years. The West Virginia State Department of Health requested the Public Health Service for assignment of another medical officer, and this was done in February 1948.

To bring the story up to date, in the last 2 years various new developments in public health administration have become reflected in the Monongalia County program. A system for public grading of restaurants has been initiated; routine serological tests for syphilis have been instituted weekly in the two local jails; a routine weekly chest x-ray clinic open to anyone has been developed; and chest x-ray examinations have been done on every patient entering the Monongalia General Hospital. A diagnostic clinic for schoolchildren has been started, and a system of teacher observation of student health has been developed. Motherhood classes are now provided for expectant women; topical fluoride dental clinics have been started; and local public health laboratory services for clinical tests are now offered. The cancer detection service has been expanded and human relations teaching is promoted in the schools. A full-time community health educator has been added to the staff of the County Health Department; a County Health Council has been organized to help coordinate all local activities relating to health; systematic nutrition service has been added to an expanded schedule of well-child conferences; and attention has been given to education on safety and accident prevention. To handle the expanded services, additional nurses and clerks have been added to the staff.

In retrospect

As these new programs developed over the years, the previously established activities were generally continued, though sometimes with lesser emphasis. Sanitary inspections regarding garbage, for example, dwindled after a publicly operated garbage disposal system was inaugurated. The entire load of communicable disease visiting, with quarantine and isolation measures, lightened as immunizations and other factors reduced the incidence of cases. In general, however, the new programs were simply cumulative, and the total volume of organized preventive services became greater each year. Not that there were no recessions. Every social movement has its ups and downs, and there were periods with temporary setbacks, as were noted. But the long-term direction was clearly toward expanded responsibilities for community health service.

From this account a few major trends in public health organization can be discerned. One is the gradual rise in responsibility, authority, and contributions by higher levels of government—first the city, then the county, then the state, and finally the federal government. Actually the higher levels have not usurped the powers of the lower levels, but they have acted as stimuli, guides, and sources of financial support for the local health authority.

Second, there can be discerned a gradually increasing concern for problems of personal health. Initial attention exclusively to the "impersonal" environment has gradually extended to include concern for individual personal health. Immunizations, well-child conferences, chest x-ray studies, VD clinics, and cancer detection examinations all represent personal health services. As a corollary, decreasing reliance is put on the force of law and compulsion and increasing emphasis on education as a means of getting results in health maintenance.

Third, there can be seen a gradual expansion of community support for and participation in organized health services. This is expressed in the launching of new health programs by various voluntary civic agencies. As these new programs demonstrate needs and prove the value of organized action, government gradually enters the same sphere and assumes responsibility. This has been seen in tuberculosis control, maternal and child health services, and cancer control. As governmental services expand, voluntary interests do not shrink, but tend to shift to other spheres, providing further stimuli all the time.

Finally, it is evident that progress is slow, and there is a considerable lag between the time that a measure may be recognized as reasonable and the time it is actually carried out. This lag is apparently caused by various sociological, psychological, and economic obstacles to change, the nature of which could only be touched upon occasionally in this historical review.[21] There can be little doubt, however, that the *rate* of development of a public health program depends directly on general public understanding of health needs. The lesson for the many counties still lacking in effective public health organization is obvious.

This historical sketch of developments in Monongalia County, West Virginia, is centered on the development of those services we now recognize as part of public health. It must be emphasized that this is only one current in the total stream of organized health activity—not to mention the story of purely private, individualistic medical practice. Some consideration has been given to public medical services for the indigent, but there are many other organized programs of health service playing a part in Monongalia County—or any other county today, the backgrounds of which have not been traced. There was the development, for example, of group prepayment plans in local industries, workmen's compensation medical care, the vocational rehabilitation program, veteran's medical services, the health plans of the lodges and fraternal orders, the charitable health programs of the service clubs, the mental and tuberculosis hospitals, the state licensure authorities for medicine and allied fields, the professional societies, and the many voluntary health or social welfare agencies, all of which have contributed to the total stream of community health activity.

The focus on public health organization alone, however, may be sufficient to show the general nature of the historical movement. We see a steadily broadened field of public responsibility for the individual's health and well-being. For those who work in the field of public health administration, faced with day-to-day problems, the process of social change may seem slow. Every new development is accompanied by greater or lesser controversies, for there is always resistance to new ideas when old ones seem to have served well. But as Heraclitus said, of one thing we can be certain—there is always change. We are in the midst of such change, of course, today. Perhaps it is because the expansion of our knowledge has been so rapid in recent decades that the lag in its social application at present seems particularly wide. A review of the past in a single rural county, nevertheless, may help to assure us that while we may never quite get to the goal we envisage in each lifetime, the expanding application of medical and sanitary knowledge, known as public health, results in the progressive enrichment of man's personal and community life.

References

1. City (Town or Burrough) of Morgantown: Council Journal, Nos. 1-20, 1838-1927.
2. City of Morgantown: Ordinance Books, Nos. 1-3, 1907-1944.
3. Monongalia County, West Virginia: Miscellaneous order books, Nos. 1-11, 1892-1929.
4. The Morgantown Post: 1903-1949.
5. The New Dominion: 1919-1928.
6. The Dominion News: 1940-1949.
7. Monongalia County Health Department: Monthly reports, 1929-1947.
8. Health Conservation Contests: General fact-finding schedule, 1941.
9. School Nurse's Annual Report to the Monongalia County Board of Education: 1934-1936.
10. American Public Health Association: Evaluation schedule, 1942-1945.
11. Personal communications from: Mr. Brooks Cottle, Miss Mary Grace, Mrs. Ethel Craig Gump, Mr. William Hart, Mr. Elmer Prince, and members of the Monongalia County Health Department staff.
12. Winslow, C. E. A.: The conquest of epidemic disease, Princeton, N.J., 1944, Princeton University Press.
13. Bowditch, H. I.: Public hygiene in America, Boston, 1877, Little, Brown and Co., p. 438.
14. Kramer, H. D.: The beginnings of the public health movement in the United States; Bull. Hist. Med. 352-376, 1947.
15. Toner, J. M.: Report of the American Public Health Association, vol. 1. In Smillie, W. G.: Public health administration in the United States, New York, 1940, The Macmillan Co., p. 15.
16. Writers' Program of the Work Projects Administration: West Virginia: a guide to the mountain state, New York, 1941, Oxford University Press, Inc., p. 129.
17. Leigh, R. D.: Federal health administration in the United States, New York, 1927, Harper and Brothers, pp. 34-37.
18. Rice, J. L.: Health for 7,500,000 people (annual report of the Department of Health, City of New York, 1937), New York, 1938, N.Y. City Dept. of Health, p. 230.
19. Rosenau, M. J.: Preventive medicine and hygiene, ed. 6, New York, 1935, Appleton-Century-Crofts, p. 438.
20. Mustard, H. S.: Government in public health, New York, 1945, Commonwealth Fund, p. 72.
21. Stern, B. J.: Social factors in medical progress, New York, 1927, Columbia University Press.

CHAPTER 3 Organized health services in a rural county

Organized programs of health service for special population groups, selected diseases, or the provision of certain technical services have evolved in the United States in bewildering variety and complexity. Most have been sponsored by agencies other than health departments, and many emanate from voluntary bodies. Within the public sector numerous governmental agencies at local, state, and federal levels are concerned.

In 1948 to 1949 the impact of these many and varied programs—curative and preventive, governmental and voluntary—on the population of one rural county was studied. No less than 155 different agencies were identified, and, considering their subdivisions in different localities, the number of discrete organizations amounted to 640. The scores of agencies are analyzed into eight types, depending on their principal means of financial support and source of authority; each type of agency, moreover, is found to be represented at local, state, and national levels, whether governmental or not. The health services provided are analyzed into nineteen distinct types of preventive activity and twenty-four categories of medical care programs.

This study was published, with the coauthorship of Ethel A. Wilson, as *Organized Health Services in a County of the United States,* Public Health Service Publication No. 197, Washington, D.C., 1952, U.S. Government Printing Office. This chapter is drawn from the "Summary and Discussion" of this monograph, pp. 76-91. Since 1952, of course, many new programs of organized health service have taken shape in America, urban and rural, but the complexity of affairs existing even more than 20 years ago may help to clarify the meaning of "pluralism" applied so often these days to the health service system or "nonsystem" of our country.

With scores of agencies engaged wholly or partially in health programs, some governmental and some voluntary, many local in sponsorship and many state or federal in authority, it is obvious that organized health services in Monongalia County are highly complex. The classification of some nineteen preventive programs, some twenty-four medical care programs, and research and training activities offered in this study may help to explain matters theoretically, but the day-to-day provision of organized health service is not nearly so orderly or logical.

The problem

The ultimate test of the effectiveness of any social action is its ability to meet the needs of an individual case. A recent experience in Monongalia County may illustrate the problems in health service.

A County Health Department nurse was called by a teacher in a rural school to investigate the home conditions of Richard, a 14-year-old boy in her class. Richard didn't seem well. The nurse visited the child's home and found Richard living with his grandfather under very poor conditions. Richard had had a rupture since infancy, but the family had been unable to afford the cost of surgical repair. Richard was referred to the County Health Department's school diagnostic clinic, where the examining physician found he needed a hernial repair, a tonsillectomy, and treatment for malnutrition.

Richard's grandfather was receiving a pension from the United Mine Workers of America Welfare and Retirement Fund (a national agency), so the nurse called the Fund's district office for assistance. Since the child's father was not a member of the miner's union, she was told he could not be helped. The County Department of Public Assistance was then approached for possible help from the State Department of Public Assistance medical care program. The resources provided by the grandfather's pension, however, were sufficient to make the child ineligible for public assistance medical services.

The nurse thereupon turned to voluntary agencies, going first to the local Family Service Association, an agency supported by the Monongalia County Community Chest. This agency indicated that their limited funds for medical aid to persons not receiving general casework service were exhausted. Not yet discouraged, the nurse contacted the county chapter of the Society for Crippled Children and Adults, the voluntary agency deriving its funds principally from the sale of Easter seals. The volunteer worker representing this agency stated that funds could be put up for the cost of the tonsillectomy, but there were not sufficient resources to finance the hernial repair.

The following day the County Health Department nurse called the head of the child welfare committee of the Morgantown Kiwanis Club. This gentleman stated that the club might be able to finance the hernial repair if a surgeon would be willing to perform the operation for a reduced fee of $25.

This required telephone calls to several physicians until one was found who was agreeable to this fee. The County General Hospital, however, required the full ward rate for its services, which were estimated to cost about $75 for this case. The Kiwanis Club was informed that the total cost, therefore, would be $100. Some days passed before the next meeting of the club's child welfare committee, at which it was decided to pay $50 toward this total cost. The committee decided also to make an independent financial investigation of Richard's family to confirm the reported medical indigency.

To secure the remaining $50, contact was made with the auxiliary of one of the American Legion posts in the county. Since Richard's father, who was now not living in the county, was not a war veteran, this group stated it could only contribute $25. For the remaining $25, the nurse made inquiries to the local women's organization, the Morgantown Service League. This organization had a special fund for preschool children and another for cancer cases, and Richard's case fell in neither category. A special meeting of the executive board of the League had to consider the matter, therefore, before it was acted upon favorably, and $25 was voted for this case.

Richard finally got his tonsillectomy and his hernial repair. The case-finding had been done by a public education agency, the diagnosis by an official health agency, the tonsillectomy was financed by one voluntary health agency, the hernial repair by a men's service club, and the hospitalization by a women's club and a veteran's organization auxiliary. Two physical defects were corrected through the persistence of a public health nurse. The correction of Richard's malnutrition and the entire social situation that led to it remained unsolved.

Richard's case is not atypical. If it is in any way unusual, it is in the determination of a health worker in following through amid the maze of organizational complexities involved in getting help for one child. Such efforts take time from a working schedule packed with other duties. More often individuals in need of health service, either preventive or therapeutic, do not get it because of the obstacles in the way or because of sheer lack of resources.

It should not be concluded that the complexities of health service organization yield only confusion. A tremendous volume of effective health service is rendered in specified categories of health need for which services have been organized. The case of Richard, however, illustrates the consequences of the high degree of health service specialization and categorization that has developed. If a human need falls precisely within some category for which group action has been taken, it may be met. But in the wide spaces between the organized pigeonholes, needs are often left unserved completely.

Another general feature of organized health services is illustrated by this case. It is that, even within the specifications of various organized programs, the quantitative resources are often meager. A crippled children's society or a men's service club may be earnestly devoted to humane objectives, but the amount of money at hand may be woefully insufficient to meet the actual needs, even in a restricted field. The partial gaps in a sphere in which some organized action has been taken may be just as serious as the complete void in a sphere in which no action has been taken.

Despite the multiplicity of agencies serving health purposes and the variety of specialized functional programs, inadequacies should not be surprising. Human health needs represent a tremendous area for social action. Although many segments of that area have been encompassed within organized programs, large sections in the field remain untilled. The concern of this study is less with the untilled portions of the field, however, than with the fruitfulness and orderliness of those sections that have been cultivated. What, then, are the principal overall findings of this study of organized health services in Monongalia County?

Summary of findings

It has been found that eight types of agency are concerned with the provision of organized health services in Monongalia County, and that these may be classified with reference to their principal source of funds. Considering only the principal varieties of organization, and not counting the several "chapters" or hierarchical divisions of each body found to have an impact on the county, there are 155 different agencies with organized health service.

These are distributed as follows:

A. Agencies supported by tax funds
   1. Official health agencies   27
   2. Other official agencies with health functions   42
B. Agencies supported by voluntary contributions
   1. Voluntary health agencies   13
   2. Voluntary social agencies with health functions   10
C. Agencies supported by economic transactions
   1. Health service enterprises   6
   2. Industry and labor with health functions   10
D. Agencies supported by individual members
   1. Professional and auxiliary organizations   17
   2. Civic and social groups with health functions   30

This summary of agencies understates the complexity of the situation since many organized functions involve several separate bodies at the local, state, or national levels. Within the county there are, for example, sixteen farm women's clubs and forty-five parent-teacher associations, although each of these is considered only one agency in the summary above. At the state level there are three separate tuberculosis sanatoria serving the county and at the national level at least ten commercial insurance companies selling "health and accident" policies to local residents. A more thorough compilation of the discrete organizations involved, taking full account of various chapters and subdivisions functioning at local, state, and national levels, is given in Table 3-1.

Agencies are, of course, only a means to a social end. An understanding of their effectiveness and their relationships to each other requires analysis in terms of their objectives. Such analysis indicates that when the multiple organized health services are described in terms of health purposes, nineteen

Table 3-1. Agencies involved in organized health service: number of discrete organizations, by type

Type of agency	Local	State	National	Total
Official health	8	21	4	33
Other official	24	17	23	64
Voluntary health	15	7	11	33
Voluntary social	74	4	6	84
Health enterprises	11	0	21	32
Industry and labor	177	1	6	184
Professional	10	11	28	49
Civic and social	128	7	26	161
All types	447	68	125	640

categories of preventive service and twenty-four categories of medical care are found. A summary of the varieties of agency involved in each preventive health program is presented in Table 3-2 and in each medical care program in Table 3-3. In these tabulations the several chapters or administrative subdivisions of an agency are counted only once, even when many such units (such as various coal mine prepayment plans within the county or various local-state-national offices of a voluntary cancer society serving the county) performed organized health services.

In Table 3-4 (preventive services) and Table 3-5 (medical care) account is taken of the various discrete organizations involved in different health programs at the local, state, and national levels. These tables enumerate the multiple chapters or administrative subdivisions of organizations for various programs. In Table 3-6 the varieties of agency involved in research and training for health service are tabulated by type, and the discrete units are tabulated by administrative level.

From these various tabulations, a few overall conclusions may be drawn. It is evident, for one thing, that a multiplicity of agencies of all four types

Table 3-2. Preventive health service programs: varieties of agency involved, by type of agency

Type of service	Official health	Other official	Voluntary health	Voluntary social	Health enterprise	Industry and labor	Professional	Civic and social	Total
Vital statistics	5	1							6
Water supply and excreta disposal	4	1							5
Milk sanitation	3	1							4
Food and drug control	4	3							7
General sanitation	3	1						1	5
Safety	1	7		2		1		5	16
Communicable disease control	5	3	1						9
Venereal disease control	3	2	2					1	8
Tuberculosis control	3	3	1	1				3	11
Maternal health	3		1			1	1	1	7
Infant and preschool health	4			1				4	9
School health	2	3	1	4			1	3	14
Nutrition	2	7	2	1	1			4	17
Dental health	3	1					1		5
Industrial and adult health	2	4				7			13
Chronic disease	2		3				1	3	9
Mental health	4	2	3					2	11
Health education	2	4	4	3	2		1	9	25
Laboratory services	2	1							3

Table 3-3. Medical care programs: varieties of agency involved, by type of agency

Type of service	Official health	Other official	Voluntary health	Voluntary social	Health enterprise	Industry and labor	Professional	Civic and social	Total
Public assistance	4						1		5
Medically indigent				3				2	5
Employees	1	1				7	3		12
Lodge members								8	8
Children	1		1	1			1	3	7
Military	1	4							5
Veterans		2		1				3	6
Students		1			1				2
Prisoners		4							4
Hospital	2	2			1		4	3	12
Physicians	3	1			1		3		8
Dental	3	1					1		5
Nursing	3						2		5
Nursing home	3	2	2					1	8
Auxiliary	4	2		1		1	3	2	13
Funds					2				2
Tuberculosis	3		1					1	5
Mental disease	2	1	1						4
Venereal disease	2								2
Crippling conditions	3	3	2					3	11
Cancer	2		1				1	1	5
Eye and ear disorders	1	1						1	3
Occupational disease		2				2			4
Disaster victims				2					2

Table 3-4. Preventive health service programs: number of discrete organizations involved, by administrative level

Type of service	Local	State	National	Total
Vital statistics	4	1	I	6
Water supply and excreta disposal	6	2	1	9
Milk sanitation	1	2	1	4
Food and drug control	1	2	4	7
General sanitation	7	2	1	10
Safety	54	6	8	68
Communicable disease control	4	5	4	13
Venereal disease control	9	1	3	13
Tuberculosis control	10	9	8	27
Maternal health	4	3	3	10
Infant and preschool health	8	2	4	14
School health	94	4	5	103
Nutrition	71	10	8	89
Dental health	3	2	2	7
Industrial and adult health	128	2	6	136
Chronic disease control	8	3	5	16
Mental health	13	3	3	19
Health education	149	15	25	189
Laboratory services	1	2		3

Table 3-5. Medical care programs: number of discrete organizations involved, by administrative level

Type of service	Local	State	National	Total
Public assistance	2	2	3	7
Medically indigent	6	1	3	10
Employees	76	3	7	86
Lodge members	9		9	18
Children	69	1	4	74
Military			5	5
Veterans	7	3	5	15
Students	1	1		2
Prisoners	6	1	1	8
Hospital	10	3	3	16
Physicians	4	5	18	27
Dental	3	3	1	7
Nursing	5	2	1	8
Nursing home	7	3	2	12
Auxiliary	7	7	8	22
Funds	8		10	18
Tuberculosis	3	5	1	9
Mental disease	2	4	1	7
Venereal disease	1	1	1	3
Crippling conditions	9	6	7	22
Cancer	4	2	1	7
Eye and ear disorders	1	3	1	5
Occupational diseases	71	1	2	74
Disaster victims	2	2	2	6

Table 3-6. Research and training programs: varieties of agency involved, by type of agency, and number of discrete organizations, by administrative level

	Research	Training
Type of agency		
Official health	2	4
Other official	1	2
Voluntary health		
Voluntary social		1
Health enterprises		
Industry and labor		
Professional		11
Civic and social		
Total	3	18
Administrative level		
Local	1	14
State	1	10
National	1	26
Total	3	50

of financial support are involved in organized health services. Multiplicity is not confined to government, private industry, or voluntary action; it is characteristic of all spheres of activity. The largest variety of agencies concerned with health are tax-supported and are engaged in general functions, to which health is incidental.

Second, multiplicity of agencies is found at all levels—national, state, and local—whether agencies are governmental, voluntary, or in the world of business. Administrative hierarchies, moreover, are by no means confined to government as is sometimes supposed, but are a feature of all types of organized action relating to health.

Third, discrete units of a particular agency tend to be most numerous, for obvious reasons, at the local level. This is most marked for voluntary agencies and private industry. Still, even at the state and national levels, several different units of a particular type of agency may be found.

With respect to analysis of functional programs, further observations may be made. Among preventive services, five or more agencies are found to be involved in every class of preventive service except laboratory services, which involve three agencies. The number of agencies concerned in fairly well-established functions, like those of environmental sanitation, tend to be relatively few; the number involved in more newly conceived programs, like health education, nutrition, and safety, are relatively great. Official health agencies are concerned with every class of preventive program, and this is true of none other among the eight types of agency.

Among medical care programs, two or more agencies are involved in each category. Every one of the eight types of agency is concerned with several categories of medical care program.

Agencies at local, state, and national levels are concerned with every class of preventive program except laboratory services. The same is true of the medical care programs for all except four categories.

The greatest number of discrete units is found for the programs serving employees of certain companies and programs involving care of occupational injuries or illness. These represent mainly different local business enterprises. Programs for children also concern many local units, representing different local chapters of parent-teacher associations or scout troops. Research activities in the county are relatively few, and training functions are primarily carried out by the professional societies.

A "counting of noses" among agencies in this way may serve to show the complexity of organized health services of every type, but it does not clarify the relative importance in total organized health service of different agencies and different categorical programs. Moreover, it does not give perspective on the contributions of different agencies within specific functional programs. To do this comparisons of the scope and content of particular programs is necessary.

Quantitative data on volume of services and costs are unfortunately not readily disclosed and not complete enough to yield summary tabulations. Nevertheless, from the data available, a few general observations may be made.

Viewing organized health services as a whole, far greater sums are spent on medical care than on prevention. Individual categorical programs such as services for veterans, workmen's compensation cases, or sanitorium care for tuberculosis involve greater expenditures than the entire appropriation for the County Health Department from all local sources. This point bears emphasis because, emanating as they do from higher levels, the impact of those programs on the community are sometimes not fully recognized by local citizens.

Among preventive programs, the greatest overall volume of services and expenditures relate to official health agencies. Other official agencies with health functions play a large role in school health services, safety, food and drug control, nutrition, and industrial and adult health. The voluntary health agencies play a major role in tuberculosis control, chronic disease control, and health education. All other types of agency, while numerous in their supportive relationship to various individual preventive programs, do not in the aggregate make a great impact in volume of services or expenditures.

Among medical care programs, the largest by far in the county are those for employees of certain companies, especially coal miners and their dependents covered in prepayment plans. Veterans constitute another group on whom relatively large sums are spent. Special arrangements for the "medically indigent" are rather meager, although this segment of the population is large at any one time. Among medical care programs for special classes of service, organized efforts for hospitalization have been greatest. Among programs for special illnesses, the care of tuberculosis has the greatest financial weight.

In programs of either preventive service or medical care, where government has entered the field for some time, the volume of its services tends to exceed the number of services provided by voluntary agencies. This is seen strikingly, for example, in the medical care programs for crippled children, where a number of voluntary agencies are at work supplemented by the crippled children's program of the State Department of Public Assistance (financed by federal and state tax funds). The services and expenditures of the latter agency exceed considerably the combined efforts of several voluntary agencies in this field. The same applies to preventive health services for schoolchildren, infants, and mothers; for venereal disease control; and dental health. In all of these fields voluntary efforts continue to play some part. The greater number of governmental services as compared to services of voluntary agencies is also seen in medical care programs for the indigent, veterans, and persons with cancer or tuberculosis—all fields in which voluntary action tended to precede official action. On the other hand, there are many spheres in which governmental action has not yet been taken or has only recently begun, and in these fields the programs of voluntary agencies or economic enterprises are of the greatest significance.

It is important to be reminded that the configuration of organized health programs in a rural county today is the result of a complex historical process, in which many separate streams of development have flowed side by side. In this connection, an historical study of the development of public health services in Monongalia County has been made,[1] tracing the rise of each of the specialized segments of the current pattern of activity of the county health department. While this study was focused on public health, rather than total organized health services, its general conclusions are relevant to the present study.*

Overlapping and gaps

With the several separate historic origins of the various segments of total organized health service, it is obvious that there must be some confusion in the impact of these programs, preventive and therapeutic, on individuals. Analysis reveals nineteen separate preventive and twenty-four separate medical care programs, but the separateness of these is largely conceptual and technical. Many different agencies may be involved within one so-called program, and the efforts of one agency may cut across many different programs. More importantly, the same individuals may be affected by several of the preventive and numerous medical care programs at the same time. With respect to the medical care programs, to quote from another paper of ours[2]:

> We can think of total medical care needs as represented by a large cube. One dimension is the population, the second is the whole spectrum of illness which people may suffer, and the third is the scope of different classes of medical and allied services available to diagnose and treat these afflictions.
>
> In a truly comprehensive . . . program of organized medical care, this cube is filled solid. In other words, all the people would be assured all classes of service for all ailments. In any community today, however, we find variously shaped islands within this cube filled in. For certain segments of the population, like members of the armed forces, all classes of service are available for all conditions. For certain ailments, like tuberculosis, the entire population is served with respect to one class of service: hospitalization. For certain classes of service, like dental care, certain segments of the population (limited usually by age level and income) are provided service for certain conditions of the teeth. Every community has its own special configuration and doubtless no two are alike. Yet the dimensions of the medical care cube are so great, that in any community typically only a minority fraction of the cubic volume is filled by organized programs.

The same sort of conceptual analysis might apply to preventive services as well. Society has developed preventive programs directed against particular diseases such as syphilis, diphtheria, or typhoid fever. There are other programs devoted to any condition in particular persons such as infants, schoolchildren, or industrial workers. There are still other programs utilizing particu-

*See Chapter 2.

lar techniques for the prevention of any condition in any person, such as vital statistics, laboratory services, or health education. A cube of preventive health services built along three axes could be constructed in any community, and various islands within it would be occupied. Only in a truly comprehensive program would the total cube of prevention be solidly filled, even if the dimensions of the cube were limited by present-day knowledge.

We hear much, in community health surveys, about overlapping and gaps among the functions of different agencies. That there are numerous gaps in Monongalia County between total health service needs and available organized programs is evident. The existence of real overlapping of functions, however, is open to question. It is true, as mentioned previously, that many different programs affect the same individuals, and many agencies may be working in the same category of service, for example, the promotion of the health of schoolchildren or the treatment of cancer. But this does not mean duplication of functions. A plotting of services in a theoretical three-dimensional graph or cube suggests that real duplication is rare indeed. The volume of total need for both prevention and medical care is so great that even when several agencies tackle the same general problem it is rare that the total problem is solved. Inevitably, whether by clear arrangement or by the natural course of events, the operations of different agencies tend to complement each other.

This can be seen in many instances. In both the prevention and treatment of tuberculosis, for example, many agencies play a part: official health agencies, voluntary health agencies, and civic and social groups—agencies at local, state, and national levels; yet each of them is directed to a different facet of the large problem of tuberculosis. Public health agencies, as well as boards of education, parent-teacher associations, women's clubs, and even the Federal Department of Agriculture through its support of school lunches, are involved in the promotion of the health of schoolchildren. All these efforts impinge on the same children, of course, but they do not constitute duplication any more than the butcher, the baker, and the candlestick maker duplicate each other when all three serve the same family.

This is not to imply that a multiplicity of agencies presents no problems. There are, indeed, many difficulties in administrative efficiency created by multiple sources of programs, even though their end results in services may not overlap. There are wastes in administrative staffs, both full-time and volunteer. This is frequently recognized in the task of fund-raising by voluntary agencies. There are losses of time and money in travel expenses, when representatives of several agencies visit the same family. There are extravagances in record systems, when several agencies keep different records on the same recipients of service. There are confusions in the relationships of different agencies to the same providers of health service in a community: the physicians, hospitals, laboratories, and others. There are irritations and misunderstandings in relationships with organized institutions such as schools, clubs, or factories, when different agencies, albeit with different objectives, make contact for various health purposes. Most importantly, there is a loss of qualitative performance when one family is contacted by many different agencies, no one of which acquires a total knowledge of the situation.

Nevertheless, far greater than the problems caused by multiplicity of agencies per se is the problem of gaps. Despite the great variety of programs, total needs are not met—not even in the fields in which a dozen or more agencies are at work. Some of these shortcomings have been suggested. Program by program, through the forty-three categories of prevention and medical care, gaps may be discerned by relating the volume of services rendered to the volume of recognized needs.

In the exposition of health functions in this investigation, evaluations of effectiveness were not made, but it is obvious that, in day-to-day affairs at the grass roots, goals are not always matched by achievements. There is often a wide gap between the declared purposes of an agency and what actually is accomplished. Examples are numerous. County Health Department nurses visit the homes of newborn infants on the basis of information from birth certificates furnished by the local registrar, but how many infants are not seen? The staff is large enough to reach only a fraction of the homes. The County and State Departments of Public Assistance finance medical services for indigent persons, but how many cases are unattended? The funds available support a volume of services much lower than are received by the general population, although the health needs of indigent persons are far greater. The factories are inspected by the State Department of Labor for accident hazards, but accidents occur. The farm women's clubs educate their members on sound dietary practices, but malnutrition is found. The Tuberculosis and Health Association and the official health agencies seek early cases of tuberculosis through many channels, but far advanced cases still appear. Instances could be offered in every field of preventive service or medical care.

There are, moreover, many spheres of possible organized health service in which Monongalia County has made virtually no headway. Some examples of services missing in Monongalia County are: a general medical and surgical clinic for the medically indigent, diagnostic and treatment services for the ambulatory with mental disorders, adequate postgraduate training for physicians and others, dental care services for moderate-income adults, prepayment for home and office medical care for nonindustrial groups, and bedside nursing services for the chronically ill in the home, to mention only a few.

Deficiencies are, of course, not unique to Monongalia County, and their evaluation is not the purpose of this study. In relation to other rural counties of comparable size and wealth, there is good reason to believe that the level of organized health services in Monongalia County is high. The question is: what is the best form of organization of those services that are now available and already having an impact on the county? No blueprint of "model organization" can be offered, but some of the factors in rational health service planning may be discussed.

Perhaps it is simplest to start with this extreme consideration: would it be best for all health service programs in the county to be administered totally and exclusively by one local agency? Presumably on such a basis maximum economy and efficiency in administration might be achieved, but to raise the question is to reveal its fallacies.

Local-state-national relationships

No organized social service in modern society can function well as an island to itself, within the boundaries of a particular county or town. Local health programs grow and improve in their scientific quality by stimulation and guidance from centers of knowledge and skill. These influences call for organization at higher geographic levels, especially state and national. Equally or more important, financial resources within a county are often insufficient to meet the needs of the persons living in that county. Yet the welfare of the nation and of the states is dependent on the welfare of each person. To apply help where it is most needed at any one time calls for pooling funds at levels higher than the community.

This applies whether the action is voluntary or governmental. The general epidemic fund of the National Foundation for Infantile Paralysis is raised nationally and used in localities of need; the Moose have their national Moosehaven for the aged and infirm; the employees of a steel company pool their monthly premiums in a mutual benefit association organized by the national corporation. In governmental programs the dependence of local units on higher administrative levels is even more compelling. As governmental social services of all types have increased, the capacities of local taxing powers to raise the necessary funds have become exhausted. Local revenues are raised chiefly from taxes on real property, and, as society has become industrialized, the source of wealth has passed from land to industrial production. State governments derive revenues from the sale of commodities like gasoline and tobacco or even from the general sales of commodities, but the possibilities of state taxes on business wealth are limited because such taxes may drive enterprises from one state to another. As a result, major taxing powers today rest with the federal government, and accordingly, major official programs of health service have grown increasingly dependent on either grants of money from the national government to the states or direct national expenditures.

It is clear, then, that organized health services today require agencies at local, state, and national levels. But what should be the relationships of these divisions to each other? Certain principles of public administration in a democracy have become axiomatic. The point of impact of any service is obviously in the local community; to do an effective job the local agency must have authority and responsibility. The local agency cannot develop the competence and civic respect required to carry this responsibility if the "parent" agency at the state or national level undertakes direct actions in the local area. The proper role of agencies at the higher level, therefore, is believed to be advisory, stimulative, and financial, while direct local actions are carried out by the local agency. Only when an effective local body is lacking should the state or national agency undertake direct actions locally.

The degree of administrative direction exerted by higher upon lower levels may vary among agencies from some, in which there are no compulsions whatever and local autonomy is complete, to others, in which all decisions are handed down from top to bottom. When programs are first initiated at a local level, such as the voluntary services of a women's club, the prepayment plan in a coal mine, the services of a dental hygienist in the school system, or the operation of a nursing home for indigent old folks, they tend to continue with a broad measure of local autonomy. When they are initiated at a higher level, however, such as state workmen's compensation activities, the National Foundation for Infantile Paralysis, the Veterans Administration, the Farm Security Administration, or the Food and Drug Administration in the federal government, a line organization tends naturally to develop in which local units, if any, mainly carry out directives from above. This comparison is somewhat oversimplified, for there are all shades of authoritarian relationships between the two extremes. Even in programs initiated locally, such as venereal disease control in the local Health Department or medical care for the indigent in the local Welfare Department, new funds from higher levels lead inevitably to some standardization of local performance according to state or national directives.

Likewise, many state and nationally initiated programs, whether governmental or voluntary, encourage local adjustments to local conditions. The impact of standards from higher level agencies has usually been for the good, since obviously greater skills can be mustered at these levels than is possible in any single local community. At the point of impact of services in a community, however, a "field command" in the actual delivery of services is probably the keynote of democratic administration. The many questions concerning the hierarchy of local-state-national relationships apply to nongovernmental as well as governmental agencies. What should the underlying relationship, moreover, be between government and the numerous agencies getting their support from voluntary contributions, economic transactions, or membership fees?

Official and voluntary agencies

There is no question about the historic role of voluntary efforts in blazing new trails of group action toward objectives in health promotion. The great advantage of voluntary action in a community, state, or nation is that it can proceed with a program on the basis of a minority decision. Governmental action in a democracy depends substantially on majority decision, and it may be many years after certain needs are recognized by a small group before the entire population is willing to act to meet those needs through government. Assurance of growth and progress in organized health services to meet all human needs, therefore, requires the permanent freedom of groups of citizens to organize.

Once a need has become fully demonstrated and a program organized to serve it, other considerations enter. Can the need always be best met by the continued operation of the independent voluntary program? Can the service be administered most economically and efficiently in this way? Can the individual be served best if certain of his or her needs are served by one voluntary agency, others by another voluntary agency, and others by many more voluntary and governmental agencies? Can providers of service do their best work by maintaining relationships with a variety of separate organizations, each interested in a particular problem?

In the nature of things there are motivations to various forms of voluntary group action beyond that of meeting health or other needs. Some speak scoffingly of the "do-gooders" in any community. While the value of an action should be judged in terms of its results rather than its inspiration, much participation in organized health service programs is undoubtedly motivated by what psychologists call substitution or compensation for personal difficulties. There can be nothing objectionable to such natural human motivations, except that they sometimes create a situation in which a program's autonomy is jealously guarded, even when the community could be served better by cooperation or integration with other programs. Because of such motivations, some voluntary groups seek extravagant publicity, out of all proportion to the impact of the group on community needs. Human factors of this type must be recognized in community health service administration.

What then is the proper role of nonofficial agencies? Obviously there is no ideal role at all times, but the functions must be reexamined at each stage of development of a community's total pattern of organized health service. Is there a point some years after the initiation of a voluntary group effort when the activities of the agency should be confined to raising funds, while the actual administration of the health services is delegated to a qualified official agency? Is there a later point when the source of funds too should be shifted to public taxes, leaving the individual citizens free to tackle some new unmet health need through group action?

Coordinated local administration

Recognizing the need for freedom of voluntary action, what should be the relationship among different official and voluntary agencies, all of which deal with the health of people in a community? Looking just at governmental agencies, is it reasonable for the State Department of Health, the State Division of Vocational Rehabilitation, the State Workmen's Compensation Fund, the State Department of Public Assistance, and the State Department of Agriculture each to maintain separate vertical staff organizations serving, among other things, various aspects of health in a county? At the federal level is it reasonable for the Veterans Administration, the Food and Drug Administration, the National Office of Vital Statistics, and the Public Health Service each to do likewise? One important instance in which separate federal agencies have utilized a common administrative outlet at the local level is the policy of both the Public Health Service and the Children's Bureau to work through the local Department of Health. Is this arrangement possible for other state and federal agencies? The same question may be applied to the scores of nongovernmental agencies providing health service.

To achieve coordinated administration at the local level, it would obviously be essential for agreements first to be reached at the higher levels. If several state or national agencies, public or private, were to utilize some common office in local communities with respect to health service, they must each be satisfied that this office is competent to assume the responsibilities involved.

There is another larger question to be faced. To what extent is it sensible to withdraw the health aspects of different overall social programs and amalgamate them? To the welfare director, health service for indigent persons is just one aspect of general welfare aid; to the school superintendent, health service for schoolchildren is just one aspect of education; to the veterans' representative, health service for veterans is just one aspect of total veteran benefits. Many of the largest organized health programs described in Monongalia County have developed as partial phases of a general activity, in which health service has had only a supportive role. This is true of agencies of all four types of financial support.

There can surely be no categorical answer to this query for all agencies at all times. If we focus attention, nevertheless, on the persons receiving service and the various providers of such service, whether preventive or therapeutic, there are compelling reasons for unification of health functions at the community level. While there are scores of different programs, they are segmented as we have seen according to theoretical concepts—diseases, techniques, or classes of person—and many different programs impinge on the same individual, many more on the same family. In one family there may be a worker covered by workmen's compensation, a child getting service from the dental program in the schools, a daughter covered by the accident insurance policy of the Girl Scouts, and a housewife learning nutrition from the parent-teacher association, and the family as a whole may get x-ray examinations from the State Health Department mobile clinic, drink milk from a dairy being supervised by the County Health Department, carry a hospitalization insurance policy sold by a local voluntary association, and receive medical care from physicians, dentists, and nurses licensed by various state authorities. This pattern of divided administration is so commonplace that we take it for granted; yet all these organized forms of social action have as their ultimate purpose the protection of the health of this family.

At the same time, the providers of health service are dealing with a score of agencies. The physician who treats an indigent person, a veteran with a service-connected condition, a worker receiving aid from the vocational rehabilitation program, a member of an industrial prepayment plan, a child assisted by the Kiwanis Club, and a patient referred from the venereal disease clinic must carry out negotiations with a half-dozen separate agencies. Each has its own rules and regulations, and none of them gets to know the physician very well because its contacts are limited to only a relatively few selected cases. In aggregate, however, all the agencies are maintaining abundant relationships with the professional personnel and institutions of the community.

If there is value in the family physician for individual health service, is there not a need for a "family physician for organized health service?" Just as medical or surgical specialists may not really duplicate each other but still may fail to treat the patient effectively because they do not see him or her as a whole, specialized agencies may also do an ineffective job. In this sphere particularly lies the challenge of coordinating prevention and medical care, so that, at the point of impingement of services on the family, prevention may be exploited to the maximum to reduce the need for medical care.

With respect to both sets of relationships, with recipients and providers of service, there is a body of complex knowledge involved. Medical science with its allied fields has become one of the most elaborate technologies in modern society. A proper organization and utilization of professional services, whether preventive or therapeutic, calls for considerable professional skill, both technical and administrative. The supply of personnel with this skill is limited in any community; it is obviously not adequate to permit separate local technical staffs for each of the separate programs reachig the people of a county. As a result, many of the programs, whether federal, state, or local in auspices, lack any qualified health administrators at the local level. The health service administration is performed by a general official, full-time or part-time, who cannot possibly possess the special health skills required, or else it is supervised by someone at a higher level, who is not acquainted with the details of health service and health needs in the local community.

The seriousness of this problem has been recognized by many agencies of public welfare. In recent years there has been a tendency for such agencies to request local public health agencies to administer medical services for indigent persons, even though these are simply one aspect of general welfare assistance. It has been recognized, too, by vocational rehabilitation agencies, which have requested administrative assistance from health departments in the supervision of the medical aspects of their program. Voluntary agencies in cancer control, tuberculosis, and other fields have done likewise.

There are financial problems created by the multiplicity of agencies, both governmental and voluntary. So long as funds are raised for special purposes, whether they are raised by taxation, voluntary contributions, economic transactions, or membership fees, they have to be spent for these purposes. Some such funds are raised locally and others are raised at state or national levels and passed along to the local community for earmarked purposes. Yet the distribution of needs in a particular community may be quite out of proportion to the composite distribution of funds. There may be relatively abundant funds available for venereal disease control, because of national legislation, but the local problem in this sphere may be small. There may be abundant funds for poliomyelitis through voluntary contributions, but the cases may be few. On the other hand, the needs in chronic disease control, dental care, or home nursing may be great, but the funds meager. Would community health needs be better met if funds from all sources, official and voluntary, national, state, and local, were allocated to some type of unified health agency in each community, which, within certain broad boundaries, would have discretion to govern the expenditure of funds in reasonable proportion to the recognized needs?

The very multiplicity of agencies tends to weaken the effectiveness of each. Inevitably there tends to be competition for funds, whether at the local, state, or national level, whether governmental or voluntary. Individual agencies are often unable to develop proper stature in community life because their scopes are limited, their staffs and funds small. There are some persons who, with an aversion to collective action, prefer things this way. They fear the amalgamation of health functions in any one agency as "empire building" and would prefer wide dispersal of functions as a protection against centralized authority. They consciously or unconsciously follow a strategy of divide and conquer. Steps toward unification of functions are sometimes greeted with the charge of "socialized medicine."

Yet the recognition of the need for coordination of community service functions in health and other fields is nationwide. Within the sphere of government there have been reorganization studies for many years. The most recent at the federal level, headed by former President Hoover, advocated a United Medical Administration, which would incorporate almost all the health functions of the many divisions and subdivisions of the federal government in one agency. Corresponding commissions in the states have made similar recommendations, such as the commission in Connecticut that proposed an expanded State Department of Health to administer health functions currently dispersed among a score of separate agencies.[3] Similar recommendations have been made in studies of other states and large cities.

At the community or county level, the growth of councils of social agencies and health councils has signalized recognition of the problem. These councils ordinarily represent both governmental and voluntary agencies, although they seldom include economic enterprises with health functions. Their goals are to promote informal coordination of services, rather than to undertake any direct administrative unification of programs. Councils of both types, it will be recalled, are organized in Monongalia County.

There are some who draw sharp distinctions among various forms of organized health activity. Governmental action is regarded as having a very different philosophical quality from voluntary charitable action, and this in turn is believed very different from action by economic interests. Yet, in the last analysis, these are all simply variations of group action to serve certain desired ends, differing mainly in the degree of participation of people in the provision and management of funds. At one end of the range are business enterprises in which services of certain types are sold to any buyer for a price; then there are membership organizations in which a group of persons pool certain amounts of money to help themselves (and sometimes others); next come voluntary agencies in which individuals give voluntarily to a fund to help those who are in need, whether or not the person has contributed; and finally there are official agencies in which everyone has been required to contribute, through taxes, and services are rendered according to the individual's need. While this may be a slight oversimplification, the element of group action is consistent throughout.

If this analysis is correct, the ultimate form of group action is found in government. If some form of unification or coordination of organized health services is sought, its effectuation may be sought most hopefully through government.

The role of the health department

In the sphere of government, the principal agency at the local level serving health purposes is generally recognized to be the Department of Health. Here, more than in any other organization at the community level, are found professional and technical skills in health service administration. Is this the logical nucleus for a broadened community agency to coordinate all organized health services at their point of impact on people?

Health departments have a long background of experience in health service administration. While their development is uneven, in all states and in the majority of cities and counties of the nation they have an established place in the structure of government. Increasingly high standards have been set for their personnel, on a merit basis. They have established, through the years, numerous relationships with various providers of health service. Their activities bring them into contact with not simply segments but with all sections of the population. They are in a position to integrate preventive and therapeutic services and, while their major emphasis in the past has been on prevention, they have increasingly been given responsibility for programs of medical care.

In Monongalia County, the County Health Department is not an isolated agency but has already achieved close working relationships with other organizations. Preventive services, such as routine chest x-ray examinations and serological tests for syphilis, are sponsored by the health department in the County General Hospital. Regular medical consultative services are provided to the district office of the State Division of Vocational Rehabilitation. Tuberculosis control activities are carried out jointly with the local chapter of the Tuberculosis and Health Association and cancer control services with the local Cancer Society. Various other relationships are maintained with the County Medical Society, the local Registrar of Vital Statistics, the Mountaineer Mining Mission, the Farm Women's Clubs, the Board of Education, the Morgantown City Council, the city police departments in the county, the local chapter of the American Red Cross, West Virginia University, and other bodies. These represent a small beginning toward coordination of organized health services. Similar relationships have developed in varying forms in other localities. Actual and potential relationships of public health agencies with programs of industrial medical care,[4] rural prepayment plans,[5] vocational rehabilitation,[6] disability insurance,[7] public medical services for the indigent,[8] and other classes of program have been described elsewhere.

It is not intended that the local health department should directly and completely operate all organized health programs in a county. Funds must come from the many agencies at national, state, and local levels in the general programs of which health services are a small part. Eligibility of certain persons for services would have to be determined by the agencies paying the bill. But at the point of actual delivery of service to the individual, or more cogently to the member of a family, a single agency should be in the picture. At the point of relationships with the various providers of service in a community, a single administrative agency should be at hand. This could well apply whether the source of funds is governmental or voluntary.

In this way, a sound overall picture of health needs could be obtained and emphasis could be placed, with certain limitations, in fields of greatest need. Qualified professional direction would be possible for all services. In fact, on this basis it might be possible to pay salaries that would attract into public health administration sufficient numbers of the most competent professional personnel in the nation. Savings on administrative overhead costs could be large. In public health nursing service the value of a "generalized program" has long been recognized, for this class of health service focuses its attention on the family unit. When the scope of service is broadened to include all preventive and all medical care programs, the values of coordinated operation would seem to be all the greater.

No attempt is made here to outline a model of coordinated health service administration in all its details. The problems to be solved in each of the forty-three preventive and medical care programs and the 640 discrete agencies described in this study would be enormous. Coordination of the dozens of prepayment plans for coal miners, for example, each of them involving a separate company, would enter the whole field of labor-management relations; yet so long as funds were collected and eligibility determined at each mine, there is no reason why all medical services could not be administered by a single health agency promoting uniformly high standards everywhere in the county. Coordination of the garbage disposal systems of the five separate towns in the county would be entirely feasible, so long as funds were contributed from each locality. The Federal Food and Drug Administration might not require a full-time worker in Monongalia County, but its local functions might easily be handled by a staff member of the Health Department, if the authority were delegated and financial support offered. Obviously additional funds and enlarged staff would be required to handle expanded functions, but these would not represent new outlays. It would be a shift of current outlays into a coordinated channel that would undoubtedly yield savings in personnel and funds.

As organized health services become more complex with new programs being added each day, it becomes all the more urgent for some integrative action to be taken. Some form of nationwide program of organized medical services for the general population has long been under discussion. If such a program should develop, a strong and effective health agency will be needed for administrative purposes in every community. Yet the tasks for such an agency need not be new, for there is no feature of a medical care program on which useful experience is not already available in the average community.

The volume and variety of organized health services found in one rural county reflect the tremendous scope of the health field, and the enormous effort of our society to bring technology and human need together through group action. A comparable study of a metropolitan community would undoubtedly yield a story even more complex. No effort has been made to compare the extent of organized services with that of unorganized or purely private health services, preventive and therapeutic. There can be no doubt that, in terms of expenditures at least, private services are today of greater importance. The trend, however, is clearly toward the gradual extension of organized services, in response to felt needs. The pattern of impact on families at various socioeconomic levels of different forms of organized health service is described in another study of a community in Connecticut.[9]

The current pattern of organized health services has grown by historical accretion of program on top of program. Although the growth of social institutions may follow certain laws, the final composite picture is not necessarily logical and practical. Yet the rule of reason cannot be applied by edict to complex social situations, and that which has grown up over the years cannot be recast overnight. The achievement of a coordinated health service administration in each community is a process that would require many years. A final pattern would never be attained, for change would never stop. The general pattern might be similar in many different communities, but details would vary. If the focus is kept on the human being served by organized health service and his or her needs rather than on the agency and the categorical program, a reasonable pattern of overall health administration may gradually be attained.

References

1. Roemer, M. I., and Faulkner, B.: The development of public health services in a rural county: 1838-1949, J. Hist. Med. 6(1):22-43, Winter 1951.
2. Roemer, M. I., and Wilson, E. A.: The pattern of organized medical care programs in a rural county, Am. J. Public Health 40:821-826, July 1950.
3. Commission on State Government Organization: The report, Hartford, Conn., 1950, Commission on State Government Organization, pp. 93-94.
4. Janis, L., and Roemer, M. I.: Medical care plans for industrial workers and their relationship to public health programs, Am. J. Public Health 38:1245-1253, September 1948.
5. Ziegler, M. E., Weinerman, R., and Roemer, M. I.: Rural prepayment medical care plans and public health agencies, Am. J. Public Health 37:1578-1585, December 1947.
6. Roemer, M. I.: A case for reciprocity, J. Rehabil., pp. 20-23, October 1949.
7. Roemer, M. I.: Opportunities for public health in disability insurance programs, Public Health Rep. 62:1657-1667, November 21, 1947.
8. Terris, M., and Kramer, N.: Medical care activities of full-time health departments, Am. J. Public Health 39:1129-1134, September 1949.
9. Roemer, M. I., and Simon, N.: The impact of organized medical services on the population of a New England town, Am. J. Public Health 42:1283-1290, October 1952.

CHAPTER 4 Health needs and services of the rural poor

In 1948, Dr. Frederick D. Mott and I collaborated in publication of *Rural Health and Medical Care,* New York, McGraw-Hill Book Company, 608 pp., as the first comprehensive account of the special health problems of America's rural population and the varied resources and programs that had been developed up to that time to cope with them.

Twenty years later, in 1968, President Johnson's National Commission on Rural Poverty invited me to report on the then current rural health circumstances, especially as they applied to the rural poor. This provided an opportunity also to determine what changes or progress had occurred in the several facets of rural health problems and services over the intervening years.

To render so large a subject manageable, it was necessary to consider only the highlights and to present them in three major parts. First are considered the health circumstances of rural life in America: the health status of rural people compared with urban, the supply and types of health personnel in rural areas, the resources in the way of hospitals and other health facilities, and the volume and types of health services actually received by the rural population. Second are considered the organized social programs designed to improve health services in the nation, including the public health programs of various types; the welfare medical services for the poor; the voluntary health insurance movement; the operation of the Medicare law of 1965 and its effects on the rural population; special governmental programs designed to help uniquely handicapped rural groups such as migratory families, American Indians, and others; further governmental health programs (in the schools, mines, etc.); and finally the efforts of other voluntary health agencies such as those attacking heart disease or cancer. Third are considered the deliberate programs designed to attract physicians and others to rural areas and the newer movements for health care regionalization and comprehensive health planning; finally there are proposed several approaches to the solution of rural health problems that may be taken at the level of the total rural economy, the national health scene, and within the bounds of local rural areas themselves.

The final report of the President's Commission was published in January 1968, with the health section appearing on pp. 311-332. The data for this review were gathered with the assistance of Daniel M. Anzel. Later, in slightly modified form, the text was reprinted as "Health Needs and Services of the Rural Poor" in *Medical Care Review* in two installments; **25**:371-390 and **25**:461-491, May and June 1968. This general account follows.

The relationship between health and social well-being is reciprocal. It has long been known that poverty causes disease, insofar as the conditions of diet, housing, occupation, and behavior associated with poverty contribute to the genesis of illness, disability, and eventually death. Rates of death and morbidity have long been highest among the lowest income groups.[1] The causative impacts of poverty on health involve both those factors influencing the biological occurrence of disease (e.g., the spread and implantation of the tubercle bacillus) and other factors influencing the procurement of health services, both preventive and curative.

On the other hand, disease has long been known to be a cause of poverty. A physically disabled person is unable to work and earn a living. On a broader scale populations decimated with malaria or intestinal parasites show lower economic productivity than healthy populations.[2] Chronic illness and its treatment may also sap the financial resources of a family, obstructing the education of its children or blighting its development in other spheres.

This reciprocal relationship between health status and social well-being or effectiveness operates in all types of geographic and social settings. Indeed, it probably applies to rural areas more than to urban, because in such areas, as we shall see, the resources for preventing and treating sickness are less developed. A specific disease or injury that has occurred, therefore, is likely to have more far-reaching social consequences for the rural patient than the same condition in an urban patient who is more accessible to prompt medical care.

Without arguing about which force may be more powerful—disease as a cause of poverty or poverty as a cause of disease—there can be no doubt about the importance of good health in the maintenance of personal happiness and community progress. There can also be no doubt about the essentiality of good medical care within a modern standard of living. Regardless of the rate of *occurrence* of disease in a population, modern social policy demands the provision of scientific and humane medical service to cope with it.

An overview of the problems of rural poverty, therefore, must examine both health needs, that is, disease and disability, and health services. The latter include the therapeutic and preventive services procured by individuals in the "open market," so to speak, and those services provided by organized social programs launched under various auspices.

Rural poverty, of course, involves two social dimensions: rurality (in contrast to urbanity) and poverty (in contrast to affluence). Whatever handicaps or, for that matter, assets, are implicit in rurality are further compounded by those implicit in poverty. This is especially true for health services for which the rural environment creates distinct obstacles that present low-income families with more difficulties within that environment. Much of the quantitative data on rural health services as well as rural health status, nevertheless, are available only along a rural-urban dimension, without further categorization of the rural *poor.* Other data are available along an economic dimension, without categorization of low-income *country dwellers.* To permit some broad understanding of the problem, however, this account of health needs and services will focus mainly on the conditions among rural populations and in rural areas as a whole. It must be understood throughout that, within this context, the characteristics of the rural *poor* are nearly always worse. Within different subjects, "worse" has different meanings, but it generally means greater deficiencies in both quantity and quality of health service.

This account will be presented in three principal parts. First, some basic background features will be drawn on health needs among the rural poor, such as health status, medical and related personnel, hospitals and other facilities, and health services received.

Second, an examination will be made of the principal organized programs now in operation to serve the health needs of rural populations, some of which follow:

Public health programs
Welfare medical services
Voluntary health insurance
The Medicare law
Migrant family and other special rural programs
Further governmental health programs
Voluntary health agencies
Attracting physicians and others to rural areas
Regionalization and comprehensive planning

Finally, suggestions will be offered on problems that must be solved.

In each of the following sections, the account will be brief, but it is hoped that the highlights will be clear.

Health status

In the early nineteenth century cities were the hotbeds of disease, mostly infectious. The rural areas, by contrast, were salubrious places, and this was reflected by marked differentials in death rates among urban and rural populations. In 1900 the annual death rate of the United States urban population was still much higher than the rural; after standardization for age-composition, it was 20.8 per 1000 urban people and 13.9 for 1000 rural people. [3]

Improvements in urban living conditions and health services have greatly reduced this differential. Rural circumstances affecting health have also improved, but at a slower rate. The result is that whatever "natural" advantages for health the rural environment may once have had, in contrast to congested cities, they have been steadily lost. By 1940 the age-adjusted urban death rate had shot down to 11.4 per 1000 per year, while the rural death rate had descended proportionately less to a level of 9.9 per 1000.

While current data for these parameters are not available (because of changing practices of the national agencies that compile health statistics), there is much indirect evidence to suggest that the distinction between overall rural and urban mortality has now almost vanished. The impact of a region's general economic development and its health technology has become so decisive that the differentials in death rates of populations are greater between the geographic divisions of the United States than between rural and urban localities as such. The lowest age-adjusted death rate in the nation in 1959 was in the west north central states (7.4 per 1000), which are highly rural, while the highest (8.5 per 1000) was in the heavily urbanized middle Atlantic

Table 4-1. Death rates by selected causes per 100,000 population per year in states of different urban-rural character, 1964*

State (percentage urban)	Chronic diseases of the aged		Conditions more readily preventable	
	Heart disease	Cancer	Accidents	Diseases of early infancy
New York (85.4%)	448.8	183.9	41.8	30.2
Massachusetts (83.6%)	395.1	167.1	41.7	23.6
Mississippi (37.7%)	301.9	128.2	70.1	48.8
North Dakota (35.2%)	330.2	134.3	63.4	33.2

*From U.S. Department of Health, Education and Welfare (HEW), Public Health Service (PHS): Vital statistics of the United States, 1964, vol. II, Mortality, Part A, Sec. 1, pp. 1-39.

states. Nearly as high as the latter, however, was the death rate (8.4 per 1000) in the east south central states (Mississippi, Alabama, Tennessee, and Kentucky), which are indeed highly rural and contain many isolated communities.[4]

Comparison of the crude death rates (i.e., not adjusted for age-composition or other elements) between states is deceptive because of marked differences in the percentages of children and aged persons in the population. For biological reasons (largely outside of social or medical control with current knowledge) the death rates of children everywhere are lower than those of old people. Thus Massachusetts, with its high level of urbanism and economic affluence, had a crude death rate in 1965 of 11.4 per 1000, compared with only 8.4 per 1000 in rural and low-income South Carolina. The principal explanation is that Massachusetts has relatively more old people and fewer children than South Carolina; with proper age adjustment, the death rate differentials almost disappear.

Among specific diagnoses, rural populations tend to have lower mortalities for the chronic diseases of later life—heart disease, cancer, and strokes—which are, indeed, the highest causes of death in the United States. They tend to have higher mortalities for the infectious and other currently preventable diseases and injuries. The epidemiological factors in back of these findings are highly complex, and any short explanation is bound to be faulty. Some comparisons for a few diseases in a few states of different rural-urban character are shown in Table 4-1. To risk an oversimplification, it would appear that the conditions of rural life reduce the risk of death for diseases that are chronic and afflict mainly the aged, while they increase the risk for infectious and traumatic conditions that with current knowledge are more readily preventable.

While the rural population still appears to hold some advantage over the urban in its record of deaths, the relationship is quite different for the burden

Table 4-2. Restricted-activity days from acute illness per 100 persons per year*

Place of residence	July 1961 to June 1962	July 1962 to June 1963
Urban	881	881
Rural nonfarm	875	881
Rural farm	894	837

*In both of these survey years, over half of the volume (as measured by disabled days) of acute illness was a result of respiratory tract disease in both urban and rural populations.[5]

Table 4-3. Prevalence of chronic disorders in different populations, 1963 to 1965

Type of area	Percent of persons with limitation of activity due to chronic illness			
	All ages	Under 45 years	45 to 65 years	65 years and over
SMSA's	10.5	4.7	17.1	43.4
Other areas				
Nonfarm	14.5	5.7	24.1	56.2
Farm	16.5	6.4	27.3	58.9

of sickness during life. The continuing National Health Survey of the U.S. Public Health Service provides a rich series of data on morbidity, based on household interviews of the noninstitutionalized civilian population.

Considering acute conditions, the urban-rural comparisons are quite variable in different years, depending on such factors as the incidence of epidemic influenza and other respiratory disorders (Table 4-2).

The comparisons for the burden of chronic disease are more consistent and, indeed, more significant. It is chronic disorder that causes the greatest overall loss of time from productive work and the greatest drain on family finances and spirit. For such disorders the prevalence is clearly higher in rural than in urban populations. Moreover, the burden is greatest in low-income families of rural areas.

Because of problems of intercensal population estimates and other considerations, the scheme for classifying urban and rural populations has changed in the U.S. National Health Survey over the years. In the latest period, July 1963 to June 1965, data on chronic illness are available by Standard Metropolitan Statistical Areas (SMSA's) (counties containing a city of 50,000 population or more plus contiguous counties that are socioeconomically integrated) and by other areas. In 1964 the SMSA's contained about 118,730,000 people who were basically urban, while the "other areas" contained about 67,065,000 people who were largely rural. The latter were divided between 55,345,000 nonfarm people and 11,720,000 farm-based people.

Using these categories, the prevalence of chronic disorders in the different populations, as of 1963 to 1965, was as shown in Table 4-3.[6] It is evident that for all ages together, as well as for each age-group separately, the proportion

Table 4-4. Disability from acute and chronic disorders in different populations, 1959 to 1961

Type of area	Restricted-activity days from all conditions per 100 persons per year	
	Males	Females
Urban	1230	1450
Rural nonfarm	1340	1610
Rural farm	1670	1710

Table 4-5. Disability from acute and chronic disorders in different populations, 1963 to 1964

Type of area	Restricted-activity days from all conditions per 100 persons per year	
	Males	Females
SMSA's	1380	1730
Other areas		
Nonfarm	1530	1880
Farm	1710	1740

of persons disabled in some degree by chronic illness is higher in rural populations, and the differential is greater for the middle and older age groups. Moreover, the burden is heaviest among farm families.

Taking a combined measure of disability from either acute or chronic disorders, the aggregate burden is also greatest among rural populations. In the period 1959 to 1961, when the older rural-urban population classification was used, the U.S. National Health Survey found the information shown in Table 4-4. In a more recent period, July 1963 to June 1964, when the SMSA scheme was used, the relative findings for overall days of disability show essentially the same relationship (Table 4-5).[7]

Analysis of the 1963 to 1964 disability data shows that under 25 years of age, and especially under 5 years, the rural record of disability is actually lower than the urban. In the more economically important working years after 25, however, and especially in males, the rural record of disability is clearly higher. In 45- to 64-year-old men, for example, the rate of restricted activity from all causes was 1980 days per 100 persons per year in the urban SMSA's, compared with 2310 days and 2730 days per 100 per year in the nonfarm and farm populations outside the urban districts.

Military Selective Service examinations provide another measure of the health status of populations, as reflected by conditons among young males. Counting all causes for disqualification, physical as well as mental disorder or mental deficiency, the national rate in 1965 was 44%. Among the twenty-five most urbanized states, the rejection rate exceeded 50% in three (Louisiana,

Table 4-6. Rate of disability as related to family income, 1962 to 1963

Family income	Disability days per 100 persons per year		
	Any restricted activity	Days in bed	Work loss
$7000 and over	1370	560	550
$4000 to $6999	1480	590	590
$2000 to $3999	1710	700	730
Under $2000	2280	970	860

Maryland, and Hawaii), while among the twenty-five most rural states, this high a rejection rate occurred in eight states (Mississippi, West Virginia, North Carolina, South Carolina, Maine, Tennessee, Alabama, and Georgia).[8] Many of these rejections reflect congenital disorders or uncorrected sequelae of past disease.

In all these indices of rural health needs, the burden is unquestionably heavier among the rural poor. In any location the rate of disability has been found to increase as family income declines. Using age-adjusted rates (thus cancelling out the bias that might be caused by the lower income of aged persons), the National Health Survey obtained the results shown in in Table 4-6 in the period from July 1962 to June 1963.

A particularly heavy burden of illness is found in members of the rural population who are black and largely concentrated in the lowest income groups. The problems of health service for nonwhite families are complicated not only by the handicaps of poverty but by the further obstacles of racial discrimination, which tend to be especially severe in rural districts.

With this bird's-eye view of health needs in the rural population and among the rural poor, we may turn to the personnel and facilities available to provide health service.

Medical and related personnel

Health status is determined by many factors in the environment, as well as in the biological reactions of the individual. The material and social environment lay the foundation for physical and mental health, but the reactions of the individual organism can be enormously influenced by the intervention of the healing arts. Physicians and a wide range of other health personnel are necessary to apply these skills.

In the rural areas of America, as elsewhere in the world, the supply of physicians and other health workers is much lower than in the cities. This has been true for at least a century, and, while certain improvements have occurred (largely resulting from better transportation), the relative deficiencies are still serious. The increasing specialization of medicine has encouraged the traditional tendency of most physicians to engage in practice in urban

Table 4-7. Physician supply (excluding those in federal employment) in counties of different urban-rural character per 100,000 population, 1963*

County group	Total	Private practice		Hospital staff, teaching, etc.	Retired
		General practice	Full-time specialty		
United States	132	35	56	34	7
Metropolitan	(143)†	(35)	(63)	(38)	(7)
Greater metropolitan‡	181	38	80	55	8
Lesser metropolitan§	133	30	62	33	8
Adjacent counties	80	38	27	10	5
Isolated	(81)	(38)	(27)	(10)	(6)
Semirural‖	87	38	31	12	6
Rural	50	38	6	2	4

*From U.S. Public Health Service: Health manpower source book, Sec. 18, Manpower in the 1960's, Washington, D.C., 1964, U.S. Government Printing Office, p. 25.
†Figures in parentheses indicate subtotals.
‡Population of 1,000,000 or more.
§Population of 50,000 to 1,000,000.
‖Contains an incorporated place of 2500 or more.

centers, where medical facilities and other technical resources are most abundant.

In 1963 there were about 42,000,000 persons in the United States living in isolated rural or semirural counties that were not even adjacent to a metropolitan county containing 50,000 people. In these sparsely settled counties there were located only 81 physicians per 100,000 population, compared with 132 per 100,000 in the metropolitan counties and those adjacent to them. The rural physicians, moreover, were mainly general practitioners, while in the metropolitan and nearby counties the vast majority were specialists in private practice or on hospital staffs.[10] The general practitioner may have certain humanistic advantages, but he or she is rarely capable of providing the soundest scientific medical service for serious illness.

The basic facts are presented in Table 4-7. It is not to be expected, of course, that every county in the nation should have the same ratio of physicians regardless of its degree of urbanization. Specialists may reasonably be expected to be concentrated in the main cities, where people should come for the treatment of complex disease problems. But the 42,000,000 people living in isolated counties, it should be realized, are a sizable distance from the cities; for the treatment of the vast bulk of their illness they must rely on the sparse supply of rural physicians in their local areas. Moreover, the low-income people in rural districts often do not have access to transportation to a distant city.

Aside from these county comparisons, whole states of predominantly rural character tend to have much lower ratios of physicians, even counting the cities within those states, than the predominantly urban states. There are twelve states with 50% or more of rural population, but only one of them (Vermont) has a physician-population ratio higher than 105 per 100,000 population. On the other hand, among the twelve most urban states (74% urban or more), all but one (Texas) has a ratio higher than 125 physicians per 100,000. New York and Massachusetts each has about 200 physicians per 100,000, while South Carolina and South Dakota each has about 75 physicians per 100,000. Over the last 25 years the ratios of physicians in all these states have improved slightly, but the proportionate state supplies in relation to each other have remained about the same.

In a few states osteopathic physicians contribute significantly to the supply of medical manpower. Over fifteen osteopaths per 100,000 population are located in Maine, Iowa, Oklahoma, Missouri, Michigan, and California. Being mainly general practitioners, these physicians are more often located in small towns and rural areas. The quality of their training, however, suggests that the service they render does not meet current scientific standards. This is much more true of outright cultists, like chiropractors, who are also settled somewhat more frequently in rural districts.

The prevailing pattern for private medical practice in the United States is the individual office, and this is especially true in small towns serving rural populations. In the larger cities physicians have increasingly come to share office facilities, and the urban "medical arts building" has promoted communications between physicians even when they are in separate quarters. The busy urban hospital is a further channel for interchange. The relative isolation of the rural or small town physician, by contrast, deprives him or her of the stimulation necessary to keep abreast of the endless advances in medical science. A slow movement toward multispecialty group practice, which is found in certain rural regions, will be discussed in a later section.

The lack of specialists in most small towns leads rural general practitioners to do more complicated surgery than their counterparts in the larger city. Bylaws of rural hospitals permit this, while in the urban centers the abundance of specialists usually results in more rigorous restrictions on the "surgical privileges" of general practitioners. This was confirmed in a recent study of several general practices in Alberta, Canada (which is much like the western mountain states), as was a finding of fewer referrals to specialists by rural general practitioners.[11]

The urban-rural distribution of dentists is even more skewed than that of physicians. In 1962 there were 54.1 dentists per 100,000 population in the United States. Among the ten most rural states, all but one (Vermont) had a ratio of under 46 per 100,000, while among the ten most urban states all but one (Texas) had a ratio of 56 per 100,000 or higher. At the extremes, there were 70 dentists per 100,000 in Massachusetts and 22.5 per 100,000 in South Carolina.[12] Small town or rural dentists, moreover, tend to have fewer auxiliary personnel (dental hygienists, aides, etc.) than their urban counterparts, and as a result their productivity per day is lower.

Nurses are extremely important in extending the arm of the physician, especially in hospitals. There are several levels of nurse, varying with their years of training, but registered nurses (RN's) are the mainstay of nursing service; they typically supervise "vocational nurses" or "nurses' aides" in hospital wards. Rural deficiencies are serious for registered nurses also, although the differentials from urban settings are less severe than for physicians or dentists. Registered nurses are mainly employed by hospitals, rather than being engaged in private practice, so that the accelerated hospital construction in rural regions, discussed on p. 77, has had a greater impact on the number of RN's in rural areas.

Although there is a generally recognized shortage of nurses in relation to the expanding demands of modern hospital service, the nurse-population ratio in the United States has steadily improved. In 1950 there were 249 registered nurses per 100,000 population, and this rose to 319 per 100,000 in 1966.[13] In rural states the rate of improvement has been even greater than in the more urban states. Mississippi's nurse supply, for example, increased from 74 to 139 per 100,000 between 1949 and 1962—a rise of 88%; New York's supply over these same years improved from 297 to 384 per 100,000—a rise of 29%.[14] The overall nurse supply in rural states, nevertheless, tends to remain lower than in urban. Much depends also on geographic region. In the New England states the supply is high even in rural Vermont, where the 1962 ratio was 429 nurses per 100,000; Texas, on the other hand, with 75% of its population urban, had a nurse-population ratio of only 170 per 100,000 in that year. Nurses who are married tend to follow their husbands in a choice of location; this is a factor that further favors settlement in the metropolitan centers.

These bare statistics on the rural-urban distribution of health personnel tell only a part of the story for the rural poor. A relatively low supply of physicians or other paramedical workers in an area means that everyone in the area is handicapped, but the poor suffer the most. If they are black they face further discrimination, such as segregation in separate waiting rooms and generally finding themselves put at the end of the queue. Even the poor whites in Appalachia or elsewhere face transportation problems in getting to a physician's office in the town, let alone traveling to a specialist in a distant city.

The training of rural health personnel, moreover, is usually more modest. Specialists in medicine, as mentioned earlier, are heavily concentrated in the main cities, and the more accomplished persons in all professions are usually attracted there. The staffing of rural hospitals must rely more heavily on "practical" or vocational nurses than on fully trained and registered nurses. The rural physician or dentist, moreover, tends to be older and, therefore, less energetic and less likely to keep abreast of new scientific advances. In a solo, as against a shared office, furthermore, he or she is seldom likely to get away for a postgraduate or refresher course. Studies in rural sections of North Carolina have disclosed the professional mediocrity that unfortunately characterizes the performance of many rural general medical practitioners.[15]

Hospitals and other facilities

Medical care of the most serious or complex illness requires hospital facilities. Twenty-five years ago, there were marked deficiencies in rural hospitals compared with hospitals in urban areas. In 1942 when there were 3.5 general hospital beds per 1000 population in the United States as a whole, the metropolitan counties had 4.7 beds per 1000, the bordering counties had 2.4 per 1000, and the nonbordering counties had 2.1 beds per 1000. In the six most urbanized states at that time there were 4.5 general hospital beds per 1000, while in the eight most rural states there were 2.2 beds per 1000.[16]

The intervening years have brought much improvement in the relative supply of hospitals in rural regions. The national population, of course, has grown a great deal over this quarter-century, and the overall hospital bed supply has risen at a somewhat faster rate, so that the national bed-population ratio in general hospitals is now 3.8 per 1000 population. However, if only "acceptable" beds under the standards of state hospital-supervising agencies are counted, the national ratio in 1965 was only 3.4 general beds per 1000.[17] The distribution of these beds among the states, moreover, is now much more even. This has been largely a result of the operations of the federal-state hospital construction program, launched under the Hill-Burton Act of 1946.

By 1965 new hospital construction, combined with a relatively greater population increase in the urban than the rural states (partly resulting from the general migration to metropolitan centers), resulted in a greater relative improvement in rural hospital facilities. Between 1948 and 1965, Mississippi, for example, had doubled its general hospital bed supply from 1.5 to 3.2 beds per 1000 population, while Massachusetts showed a decline from 3.9 to 3.7 beds per 1000. Examining the 1965 hospital bed ratios in sets of ten states by increasing degrees of rurality, the comparative urban-rural regional bed supply has been nearly equalized, as shown by the following figures:[18]

Sets of ten states by percentage rural	General hospital beds per 1000 population
11.4-25.1	3.86
25.5-33.4	3.79
34.3-41.7	4.09
43.2-52.5	3.59
55.5-64.8	3.62

Adequacy of hospital care, however, cannot be measured solely by the quantity of beds. In general, smaller hospitals are less well staffed with technical personnel and less well equipped, and it is to small-sized hospitals that rural people must usually go. Hospitals in small towns, moreover, seldom have rigorous policies for medical staff organization, so that they are less likely to meet the quality standards of the Joint Commission on Accreditation of Hospitals. In rural Arkansas, for example, only half (thirty-nine) of the eighty hospitals listed by the American Hospital Association in 1960 were accredited, and in Montana only twenty-seven out of sixty hospitals were accredited. By contrast, in urbanized Delaware thirteen out of the sixteen hospitals were accredited, as were nearly three-quarters (fifty-two) of the seventy-one hospitals in Connecticut.[19]

Of special significance to the rural poor is the sparsity of organized outpatient departments in small-town hospitals. For centuries, hospitals in the main cities have offered "free" or very low-cost medical services to ambulatory patients of low income. Partly from the charitable tradition of the hospital and partly to provide teaching resources for medical students and interns, large city hospitals have long conducted a variety of outpatient clinics for the indigent and medically indigent. Physicians using the hospitals for inpatient care of their private patients have staffed these clinics without remuneration. In small-town hospitals, however, such organized outpatient departments are seldom found. There may be an "emergency room" where anyone can come without an appointment, but this does not meet the need for regular medical care, especially for chronic ailments, among the poor.

Institutional care of the aged and chronically ill is provided increasingly in nursing homes and related "extended care facilities," as distinguished from general hospitals. These are predominantly small units (mainly under fifty-bed capacity) operated by private proprietors, rather than nonprofit agencies. Many of these facilities are simply old converted houses, in which ten or twenty aged patients are accommodated. Nationally almost 50% of their patients are recipients of public assistance.

The supply of nursing home beds tends to be lowest in the states and counties of lowest per capita income, and also where the proportion of the population in the over-65 age group is smallest. Thus, the lowest ratios of nursing home beds providing "skilled nursing care" (under 0.50 such beds per 1000 population) are found in North Carolina, Alaska, Alabama, Arizona, and Georgia. The highest ratios of beds (over 4.0 per 1000) are found in New Hampshire, Massachusetts, Vermont, and the state of Washington.[20] The rural-urban discrepancies in these institutional resouces are evident, but they are reflected less in the bed-population ratios than in the types of facilities. The best quality nursing homes are those operated by church groups and other nonprofit agencies; such facilities are typically built at the suburban fringes of the metropolitan centers. In the isolated rural counties, extended care is dependent almost entirely on small proprietary units of the humblest quality.

One important type of health facility, hospitals for the mentally ill, is provided mainly by state governments. In each of the four most urbanized states of the nation (New Jersey, Rhode Island, California, and New York) the ratio of mental hospital beds "acceptable" to the state-supervising agency exceeds 3.0 per 1000 population. In each of the four most rural states (North Dakota, Mississippi, Alaska, and West Virginia), the ratio is lower than 3.0 per 1000.[21] Examining the nation as a whole, however, the relative deficiencies in the more rural states are not so striking. In fact, mental hospitals are often used as a last refuge for senile patients who, because of poor family circumstances, cannot be cared for at home; the low-income rural states, therefore, have been relatively energetic in building mental hospitals to cope with this problem. Georgia and Virginia, for example, operate higher ratios of mental hospital beds than Connecticut and Massachusetts.

The deficiencies in this sector are reflected mainly in the staffing of mental hospitals. Everywhere in the nation these hospitals are understaffed and underequipped, but especially in the lower-income rural states. Senile and other psychotic patients from rural areas must usually go to seriously substandard facilities. This is a special misfortune for the rural poor, since everywhere mentally disturbed patients of lower social classes are more likely to be handled through institutionalization than persons of higher social rank with the same diagnosis.[22]

Thus, in summary, the total health facilities in rural regions, while they have improved over the last quarter-century, are still somewhat lower in quantity than those serving large city populations. Their qualitative deficiencies are more serious. Of course, rural patients may and do travel to distant cities for hospital care, but this is done mainly by those of moderate or high income. The financial means and the medical sophistication required to obtain medical or surgical attention in a distant city hospital are seldom found among the rural poor. It is for this reason that efforts have been made to develop networks of interrelated hospitals in large geographic regions, a subject to be discussed later in this report.

Health services received

With these deficiencies in health personnel and facilities serving rural populations, it is to be expected that the volume of services they receive would be lower than that for city dwellers. This is especially true for the rural poor, in spite of their higher burden of sickness and disability.

Medical care is obtained through private purchase, voluntary insurance, and governmental or charitable sources. In 1961 the average urban family spent $355 for all medical services, a figure that included $91 in health insurance premiums. Rural farm families, which were on the average larger, spent $310 in that that year.[23] Support for medical services by way of government, as we shall see, is also lower in rural areas.

The best measure of the day-to-day medical care people receive is the rate of contact with physicians or dentists per person per year. These contacts

Table 4-8. Medical and dental services by place of residence, 1963 to 1964*

Contacts per person per year	Standard Metropolitan Statistical Areas (SMSA's)	Outside SMSA's	
		Nonfarm	Farm
Physician's visits			
Males	4.2	3.7	3.0
Females	5.4	4.8	3.7
Dental visits			
Males	1.7	1.0	0.9
Females	2.0	1.4	1.0

*From U.S. National Health Survey. In U.S. Department of Commerce: Statistical abstract of the United States 1966, Washington, D.C., 1966, U.S. Government Printing Office, p. 66.

may take place in the physician's office, the patient's home, or in an organized clinic, but the great majority take place in an office. The basic findings for 1963 to 1964 are shown in Table 4-8. For both sexes the rate of contact with physicians and dentists is appreciably lower in the nonmetropolitan areas, farm and nonfarm. Other tabulations show that this holds for each age group, but the differential is particularly great for the very young. Differences are also greater at the lower income levels.

Hospitalization presents a different urban-rural comparison. Hospital care, more than ambulatory health care, has been supported by public funds, such as in the programs of welfare departments, the Veterans Administration, or the Indian Health Serivce. Inadequacies in physician's care of the ambulatory patient, moreover, often result in an illness becoming aggravated, so that hospital admission becomes urgent. Furthermore, physicians in rural districts who are hard-pressed for time cope with the pressures by hospitalizing patients more readily, sometimes for conditions that could ordinarily be treated in the patient's home or the physician's office. As a result of these factors, the volume of hospitalization received by rural people is not lower than that received by metropolitan area residents, unless they are actually farm families. The basic findings of the National Health Survey for the 2-year period from July 1963 to June 1965 were as follows:[24]

Type of area	Hospital discharges per 1000 population per year	Average length of stay (days)	Hospital days per 1000 population per year
SMSA's	122.2	8.8	1075
Outside SMSA's			
Nonfarm	145.0	7.6	1102
Farm	111.7	6.8	760

If the net measure of hospital days per 1000 persons per year is used, the overall rate of service to nonmetropolitan populations is lower than that to the residents of cities and their environs (these measures are, of course, by the person's place of residence rather than by hospitalization). In fact, in 1959, when the National Health Survey analyzed its data according to the older form of rural-urban breakdown, the aggregate days of hospitalization per 1000 persons per year were:

Urban	901.6
Rural nonfarm	800.0
Rural farm	704.7

As one can gather from the previous sections on medical personnel and facilities, the type of physician's care received by a country dweller is more likely to be that of a general practitioner than a specialist. In the drugstore he or she is more likely to purchase a self-selected or patent remedy, as distinguished from a prescribed medication. In the dental chair he or she is more likely to have extractions of neglected teeth than fillings or other services to preserve the teeth.

Aside from the physical handicaps of poverty, the lower level of education of rural people, especially the poor, means that they are less likely to observe principles of hygienic living. They are less likely to obtain preventive immunizations, to have prenatal care during pregnancy, to eat a nutritionally balanced diet, and to obtain periodic health examinations for early disease detection. In the poorest rural families suffering discrimination on racial or ethnic grounds, a certain fatalism and despondency may develop so that medical attention is sought only when health problems become desperate.

Public health programs

The previous pages have summarized the health status of rural people, the general resources in personnel and facilities available to them, and the medical services they receive, primarily in the "open market." There are many organized health programs in America, however, designed to protect the health of populations and to make medical care more accessible to them. The extent and character of these programs in rural areas must be examined, starting with the activities of public health agencies.

Historically, public health departments, like hospitals, had their beginnings in the largest cities; it was not until 1911 that a local public health agency was organized by a county government, with specific orientation to a rural population. Since then, about 80% of the 3071 counties in the United States have come to be served by organized health departments with full-time health officers.[25] In many sparsely settled regions, however, a "health district" composed of several adjoining counties is the jurisdictional unit.

The traditional services of public health agencies include supervision of environmental sanitation, control of communicable diseases (isolation of cases, immunizations, etc.), promotion of maternal and child health, and health education. As tools for these objectives, the departments collect vital statistics,

Table 4-9. Public health nurses in states ranked by order of rurality, 1964*

Sets of ten states by percentage rural	Population	Public health nurses	Public health nurses per 100,000 population
11.4-25.1	75,427,000	16,441	21.4
25.5-33.4	50,821,000	8827	17.4
34.3-41.7	24,940,000	3563	14.3
43.2-52.5	23,091,000	2981	12.9
55.5-64.8	18,735,000	2217	11.7

*From American Nurses' Association: Facts about nursing 1966, New York, 1966, American Nurses' Association, p. 28.

operate laboratories, and conduct clinics. In the last 25 years some health departments have broadened the range of their activities to include such programs as dental service for children, accident prevention, operation of treatment programs for crippled children, promotion of mental health, early detection of chronic noncommunicable diseases such as cancer or diabetes, and sometimes the administration of public hospitals.

These wider-ranging public health programs, however, are usually conducted by agencies based in the larger cities. Rural county or district health departments tend to carry out relatively narrow programs. Aside from the conservatism of rural county governments, the staffing of county departments is usually so frugal that there is little time for innovations. The same applies to most state health departments in the more heavily rural states. In such states the public health agency is often dominated by the state medical society, which tends to inhibit extension of governmental programs. Many of the rural county health departments, moreover, are directed by semiretired physicians who are seeking an easier life and are not inclined to move out and blaze new trails for public health improvement. It is common, moreover, for the health officer position to remain vacant for months or years when a former director has left or died. In Arkansas, for example, twenty-one of the twenty-seven local health units were without a full-time health officer in 1964, as were eighty-three of the 121 units in Kentucky. California, on the other hand, had such medical vacancies in only two of its sixty-one local health units, and in New York only three of its forty-two units were vacant.

A good indicator of the adequacy of public health services is the ratio of public health nurses to population in a state. The public health nurse is involved in most of the clinical programs (child health services, venereal disease, tuberculosis, dental care, etc.), in visiting families at home, giving immunizations in schools, offering health education, and generally acting as the foot soldier of the public health army. In Table 4-9 the ratio of public health nurses to population in sets of ten states ranked in sequential order of their rurality can be seen; it is evident that in the more rural states the ratios are consistently poorest.

Nevertheless, the operation of public health agencies in any state tends to offer special benefits for the lower income groups. In the rural South, where private health services are beyond the reach of many black families, public health clinics help to meet certain needs. Prenatal visits to public health clinics, for example, may be correlated with the births occurring in a state; in 1965 such visits were made by mothers at the rate of 186 per 1000 births in Mississippi—and at the rate of 163 per 1000 in North Carolina. In urbanized New York in 1965 the rate was only 21 per 1000 and in Pennsylvania 24 per 1000.[26] Most pregnant women in the latter states are doubtless given prenatal care by private physicians, so that the total rate of prenatal services from all sources is almost certainly higher there. But the impact of public health agency services in rural states is obviously helpful in the face of inadequacies of private medical care for the low-income population.

Welfare medical services

Another important health program specifically focused on the needs of the poor is the system of welfare agency services that include certain types of medical care. Some of these services are given in municipal or county hospitals operated directly by government, other services are purchased by the welfare client with his or her cash allotment, and still others are obtained through so-called "vendor payments" by the welfare department to private physicians or hospitals that render care to the indigent person. An elaborate set of "categories," moreover, defines persons whose financial aid and medical care are supported largely by federal grants to the states—mainly the aged poor, the poor families with "dependent children" (because of lack of a breadwinner), and the indigent blind or totally disabled. Other indigent persons requiring medical care must depend entirely on state or local funds for "general assistance."

In general the proportion of persons receiving some form of public assistance is higher in the low-income states with greater percentages of rural population. This is especially true for old-age assistance; in Georgia, for example, 28.7% of all persons over 65 years of age received such assistance in 1965, while in New Jersey it was only 2.2% of such persons. This is partly a result of the greater extent of poverty in the more rural states and partly the lesser coverage of the federal old-age insurance program (commonly known as "social security") in those states.

The financial, as well as the medical, benefits per indigent person, however, tend to be decidedly lower in the more rural states. In the program for aid to families with dependent children (AFDC), for example, the expenditures for vendor payment for medical care in the month of December 1965 were $4.84 per recipient in New York, $7.81 in Connecticut, and $6.42 in Hawaii, which is 76% urban. By contrast, the vendor medical payments per AFDC recipient in the same month were $2.53 in North Carolina, $1.35 in Maine, and $1.39 in Virginia. Moreover, in several rural states such as South Dakota and Mississippi, there was no vendor payment program at all for AFDC families; the medical care of these families had to be financed entirely from their cash allowances or obtained through the charity of physicians or hospitals.[27] A comparable differential applies to the aged poor who may obtain medical care either through the program of old-age assistance (OAA) or the special programs enacted in 1960 on medical assistance for the aged (MAA).

As mentioned earlier, rural people of low income are less accessible to outpatient clinics of hospitals than the urban poor. Yet the poor who do not fit under one of the federally aided categories (for example, a nondisabled man under 65 years of age) cannot ordinarily get welfare support for care from a private physician; they must either impose on the kindness of the physician or seek local "general assistance," which is seldom available for medical expenses outside the hospital. Although there is much talk of the "medically indigent" (i.e., those who cannot afford medical costs, although not poor enough to be eligible for public assistance), no significant governmental assistance was available for such persons before the MAA program of 1960 and the Social Security Amendments of 1965 known as "Medicare."

Under Medicare, Title XIX, there will doubtless be improvement in the support of medical service for the rural poor, although much will still depend on the ability and willingness of state governments to put up money that can be matched by federal grants. Prospects under this new law will be considered in a later section. Until now, the range of welfare medical benefits for the rural poor has been meager, limited largely to hospitalization of emergencies or severe diseases.

Voluntary health insurance

For those who are self-supporting, a major device for facilitating medical care is health insurance. Through pooled periodic payments into a fund, individuals and families gain protection against the cost of hospital or medical services, so that access to those services is greatly enhanced. There is abundant evidence that persons with health insurance receive greater volumes of medical care at all family income levels than those without.[28]

However, the rural population, especially the rural poor, suffers a disadvantage in this sphere, too. Hospitalization insurance is the most extensive form of health cost protection carried in the United States. At the end of 1965 about 80% of the civilian population had such coverage.[29] The enrollment of rural people compared with urban is appreciably lower, and the differential is even greater with respect to insurance for physician's care. Comparative data are available for 1962 to 1963 and are shown in Table 4-10. At this time the national coverage of hospitalization insurance was 70.3% according to the U.S. National Health Survey, while it is evident that among the rural poor (under $4000 family income) for both farm and nonfarm population it was less than 50%.

Table 4-10. Health insurance coverage: percentage of the rural and urban population protected by hospitalization insurance, 1962 to 1963*

Family income	Urban	Rural nonfarm	Rural farm
$7000 and over	88.8	85.3	71.2
$4000 to $6999	81.4	75.1	65.3
Under $4000	47.6	41.6	37.4
All incomes	74.5	63.8	50.8

*From U.S. Public Health Service: Vital and health statistics: health insurance coverage July 1962 to June 1963, Washington, D.C., 1964, U.S. Government Printing Office, p. 9.

The explanation of this rural handicap is not difficult. Aside from lower incomes, which, in both urban and rural sections mean less insurance coverage, rural populations are less readily enrolled in health insurance plans for administrative reasons. The great bulk of insurance enrollment is done through organized groups of people—mainly the employees in a firm or other place of work. Larger groupings are more easily enrolled than small ones. In small towns and agricultural regions, however, it is obvious that such organized groupings of people are both fewer and smaller.

Among rural nonfarm people, mine workers and their families have achieved fairly good health insurance coverage, largely through the collective bargaining of their labor unions. The Welfare and Retirement Fund of the United Mine Workers of America has provided insured hospital and specialist services with careful quality surveillance to several hundred thousand miners and their dependents since 1948.[30] The farm organizations in some areas, including the Farmers Union, the Farm Bureau, and the Grange, have also achieved the benefits of group enrollment of their memberships.

Many of the lowest income people in rural areas, however, are not attached to mining employment, to farm organizations, or to other organized groups. Their isolated status presents not only greater obstacles to health insurance enrollment in voluntary plans, but also deprives them of the financial advantage of premium-sharing by an employer. In most industrial populations the latter "fringe benefits" have been achieved over the years in labor-management negotiations.

Another result of isolation is the necessity of rural people, who do seek health insurance coverage, to depend on those policies that are sold specifically for individuals, as distinguished from groups. Because of actuarial consid-erations in the insurance business, high sales costs, and profit incentives, individual health insurance policies tend to cost more and give less. Their premiums are higher and their benefits are more restricted than those of group insurance policies. In fact, such individual enrollee policies are sold mainly by commercial carriers, and the cost-benefit ratio (i.e., the percentage of premiums paid out in benefits) is generally poorer.[31]

The great predominance of commercial health insurance coverage in rural populations is reflected by data from the separate states. In 1962 (when about

70% of the national population had hospitalization insurance), the overall distribution among the three main forms of insurance organization was as follows[32]:

Type of carrier	Percentage of enrollment
Commercial companies	56.1
Blue Cross-Blue Shield	39.3
Other independent plans	4.6
All carriers	100.0

In the more urbanized states the Blue Cross-Blue Shield and the independent plans tend to have greater proportionate enrollment, while in the more rural states the commercial companies tend to have an even greater share of the total enrollment. Thus in heavily urbanized states like New Jersey, Rhode Island, New York, Massachusetts, Hawaii, Utah, Colorado, Ohio, and Pennsylvania the commercial share of health insurance coverage is under 50%. It is over 60% however, in more heavily rural states like North Dakota, Mississippi, Alaska, West Virginia, Vermont, South Dakota, North and South Carolina, Arkansas, Idaho, Montana, Nebraska, and others.

One of the more promising developments in the health insurance field is the establishment of plans providing more comprehensive benefits than the large commercial or Blue Cross-Blue Shield entities. The health services offered under these latter organizations are mainly confined to hospitalization and physician's care in hospitalized illness; comprehensive physician's care in the home and office (or clinic) as well as the hospital is only meagerly provided. Moreover, the benefits for even hospital-based services are predominantly on an indemnification basis, with the patient usually being obligated to pay a balance of charges beyond the limit of the indemnity allowance. By contrast, a small but important share of the national population (about 4%) is enrolled in health insurance plans, usually sponsored by consumers or industrial firms, which offer comprehensive medical and hospital services. Most of these people are in plans that have physicians organized in group practice clinics.

The largest of these comprehensive prepaid medical care plans are in New York (Health Insurance Plan of Greater New York) and California (Kaiser Foundation Health Plan), and they cover essentially urban populations. In those two states enrollment in comprehensive insurance plans reaches nearly 8% of the population.[33] There are certain rural regions, however, where this type of plan has shown vitality, even though the percentage of population reached is still very small. One of the earliest was the Farmer's Union Hospital Association with its prepaid community clinic, which was started at Elk City, Oklahoma in 1929. In rural sections of Texas, Arkansas, South Dakota, Alabama, Kansas, Minnesota, Missouri, Oregon, and Washington, somewhat similar health plans are operating. Their importance is to be measured less in terms of the numbers of rural people enrolled, which are still small, than in their demonstration of sound medical service patterns, which may suggest blueprints for the future.

The voluntary health insurance movement in America has made great progress against much early opposition in enabling people to get needed medical care. Its value has been not only in lightening financial loads on families, but also in laying foundations for improvement in the quality of professional care. There is still a long way to go, however, before health insurance protection achieves its full potential of both population coverage and scope of medical benefits. Its impact so far has been less among rural than among urban people, and the very least among the rural poor. An important step forward in helping low-income people, both rural and urban, was taken by the health insurance amendments to the Social Security Act of 1965, and they will be reviewed in the next section.

The Medicare law

The provisions of the Medicare amendments to the Social Security Act of 1965 are too well known to review here, but their relative impact on rural people may be considered. First of all, with the focus on the health care of the aged 65 years and over, the benefits must be somewhat less for rural residents, since the latter include a smaller proportion of aged persons and a larger proportion of children. The national urban population (1959) has 9.3% of aged persons compared with 8.0% in the rural population.

Second, there is the problem of rural enrollment. The benefits of Title XVIII on health insurance of the aged include Part A for hospital and related services and Part B for physician's care and other special services. Part A benefits are automatically available to virtually every senior person in the nation, but Part B benefits require voluntary enrollment by the individual, with payment of a share of the premium costs ($3 per month in 1967). By January 1967, some 93% of all aged persons in the United States had voluntarily enrolled in Part B and were therefore entitled to insurance for a fairly wide range of physician's services and certain other benefits.[34]

Among rural aged persons, however, the enrollment for Part B benefits was clearly lower than the national average. Among the ten most urban states, all ten aged populations were enrolled in the Part B program at a rate higher than the 93% national average; among the ten most rural states only three of the aged populations had enrolled at a rate exceeding the average. For example, in the two most urban states (New Jersey and Rhode Isalnd) the enrollment was 96% and 95% respectively, while in the two most rural states (North Dakota and Mississippi) it was 92% and 85% respectively. These apparently small differences, a result of difficulties in communication with isolated and poorly educated aged persons in rural areas, may make a large difference in the medical care received by these noninsured persons.

A third problem in the rural operations of Medicare relates to the Civil Rights law, which requires that participating hospitals and "extended care facilities" must practice no policy of racial segregation in rendering services. About 95% of the licensed general hospitals in the nation have complied with these requirements, but those that have not are concentrated in the rural states of the South; many aged persons in those states, therefore, both blacks and whites, are being denied access to facilities for hospital care to which they are legally entitled.

There are other deficiencies in the Medicare law that are bound to strike the rural aged harder than the urban aged. Various deductibles and cost-sharing requirements naturally create greater obstacles for the impoverished aged persons found more frequently in rural areas. The practical availability of all the benefits, moreover, depends on the supply of medical and related personnel, which we know is lower in rural districts.

In spite of these weaker benefits, there can be no doubt that the social insurance principle in Medicare Title XVIII has been a boon to the rural aged and constitutes a long step forward for medical care. This new law has corrected many of the deficiencies of voluntary health insurance in rural and urban areas alike.

Another feature of the Medicare amendments is the provision for improved services for the indigent, old and young, legislated under Title XIX. As reviewed earlier, these are largely limited to certain "categories" among the poor, but the new law permits federal matching of state funds for "medically indigent" persons of the same demographic characteristics, even if they are not receiving cash assistance. This will doubtless be of special value for low-income rural people who are "categorically linked," particularly the children in families with a missing breadwinner. By 1975, moreover, the Medicare law requires that *all* medically indigent persons in a state, even if not categorically linked, must be eligible for some medical assistance if the state is to receive federal support for any of its poor residents.*

It is still necessary, however, for the states to put up approximately half the cost of this medical care for the poor, and the economic potential in the rural states remains lower. The law's requirement of a greater share of financing from state, as opposed to local, governments is, it is true, a special advantage for the residents of rural counties within any type of state. As of January 1967, however, twenty-three of the fifty states had not yet implemented the Title XIX program; of these twenty-three, sixteen were in the most rural half and only seven in the most urban half of the nation's fifty states.[35] There is much leeway left, moreover, on the scope of health services that a state may provide for its welfare beneficiaries. Hospital, nursing home, and physician's services are mandatory, but dental care, physical therapy, and drugs

---

*In the early 1970's this provision of the original Medicare law was repealed.

are optional, and these may be expensive items. There is every likelihood that this range of services for Title XIX beneficiaries will be narrower in the more rural states, and the criteria for eligibility of the "medically indigent" will be more rigid.

The Medicare law, nevertheless, constitutes a solid step forward in medical services for both the rural and urban poor, by reason of both Titles XVIII and XIX. Amendments in the coming years may well improve its provisions further.

Migrant family and other special rural programs

For certain sectors of the rural population, special programs of health service have been organized, and these must be examined briefly. Of principal current importance are migrant agricultural families, American Indians, and residents of the Appalachian region.

In the 1930's and early 1940's, when the nation was plunged into a massive economic depression, the rural areas were hit especially hard, and numerous assistance programs were developed under the U.S. Department of Agriculture. Perhaps the most imaginitive was that of the Farm Security Administration (FSA), which had many facets, including special health service programs for low-income farm families and migratory farm workers. At their peak in 1942, special federally subsidized prepaid medical care plans for FSA-borrowers reached over 600,000 persons in 1100 rural counties. In addition, about 150,000 persons in migratory families were served by special clinics or health centers established at 250 locations of seasonal labor concentration.[36] This terse summary cannot possibly convey the boundless work, ingenuity, and dedication that went into the development and operations of these remarkable rural medical care programs.

With the end of World War II, there was a retrenchment in federal assistance programs of the U.S. Department of Agriculture and a return of responsibilities to the states and counties. In most states governmental agencies did not take up the challenge in the field of health services, so that these publicly supported programs were, in effect, abandoned. The health needs of low-income farm families and migratory agricultural workers were left to be met by the traditional local welfare programs or through the private sector. Experiences of the FSA and related pioneering rural health programs, however, left their mark on the nation, especially in a heightened appreciation of the special problems of rural medical service. Enrollment of farm people in Blue Cross plans through their farm organizations, founding of some voluntary rural medical cooperatives, strengthening of rural county health departments, and the whole concept of hospital regionalization under the Hill-Burton Act were among the long-term benefits.

Health services for migratory agricultural families remained an especially vexing issue, since, being nonresident in most of the areas where they do seasonal work, these low-income people have usually been ineligible for medical assistance from the local welfare department or local public hospitals. The plight of these unfortunate adults and children, immortalized in John Steinbeck's *Grapes of Wrath* (1939), seems to be rediscovered every 20 years or so. In 1962 the federal Migrant Health Act (PL 87-692) was enacted, reestablishing federal assistance for health services to migrant workers and their dependents. Instead of a direct federal operation, however, this program authorized grants by the U.S. Public Health Service to state and local agencies (mainly health departments) for services to migrant families.

The 1962 law emphasized grants for "family health service clinics"—a politically palatable identification for general ambulatory medical care, as distinguished from the restricted preventive services conventionally offered by rural county health departments. By 1965 grants had been made to sixty local projects for such broad-gauged clinics and for other purposes including health education, sanitation, or public health nursing in twenty-nine states and Puerto Rico.[37] Undoubtedly these projects improved the health care of several thousand migrant families, among the estimated 2,000,000 such persons in the nation.

The total appropriation for these migrant health grants in 1965, however, was only $3,000,000. A study of the problem by the American Public Health Association suggested that an "average" level of medical service for these families would cost over $100,000,000 per year.[38] Exact accounting of financial needs, in relation to private resources for health care, is extremely difficult to make, but it is evident that by almost any criterion this program's impact must be small. The drop in the bucket that it offers is less important than its value in keeping alive social concern for the migrant family, whose health problems require more basic rural actions in order to be solved.

Another distinct rural population for which government has taken substantial responsibility is that of the American Indian. Of the 552,000 Indians counted in the 1960 census, about 380,000 are entitled to health services from a special network of hospitals and health centers operated by the Division of Indian Health of the U.S. Public Health Service. These are predominantly rural people, of low income, concentrated on Indian reservations in twenty-three states. The largest numbers are in Oklahoma, New Mexico, and Arizona.[39]

With origins going back to War Department treaties with Indian tribes in the early nineteenth century, the Indian health service program was operated by the U.S. Department of Interior from 1849 to 1955, and since then by the U.S. Public Health Service. Today there are forty-seven general hospitals and three tuberculosis sanatoria (from fourteen to 400 beds) earmarked for these rural people. There are about 300 field health stations attended by physicians or nurses, and, in areas of sparse Indian settlement, there are contractual arrangements for services from some 200 other local hospitals, 400 private physicians or dentists, and eighteen state and local health departments. A reflection of this program's amplitude is its expenditure for health service in 1964 of almost $138 per capita, an amount only slightly lower than the per capita health expenditure of the entire U.S. population at the time.

The outstanding feature of the Indian health service is its comprehensiveness, combining all the usual preventive services and a full range of ambulatory and institutional services for treatment. No other population group outside of the active military forces receives such wide benefits at federal government expense. As a result, the record of health improvement among Indians in recent decades is impressive, in spite of seriously impoverished living conditions. Their life expectancy increased by eleven years between 1940 and 1962, although it is still eight years below that of the average American. It is interesting to observe the daringly "socialized" patterns by which health services have been organized for this special social minority, in contrast to larger sectors of the rural poor in America.

A third group among the rural poor for whom government has taken special action are the residents of the Appalachian mountain region. In 1965 the federal Appalachian Regional Development Act (PL 89-4) was passed to help improve the conditions of life for low-income rural people in Kentucky, Tennessee, West Virginia, and western sections of Virginia and North Carolina. This program included $21,000,000 for grants to build and equip hospitals, diagnostic and treatment centers (i.e., units for ambulatory patients), and other health facilities in this region.[40] Along with this construction subsidy has gone technical consultation from the U.S. Public Health Service to help improve the basic public health and hospital services available to these mountain people.

There are other governmental health programs serving selected rural populations, like the families of personnel working for the Tennessee Valley Authority or residents of the Virgin Islands and U.S. trust territories in the Pacific Ocean. Altogether, however, these along with the three special programs described above reach only a small proportion of the rural poor in the nation.

Further governmental health programs

A variety of other governmental health programs for certain demographic groups or special diseases operate throughout the United States and have some impact on the rural poor.

Schoolchildren everywhere have the benefit of limited health protection, including physical examinations and first aid, as well as health education in the classroom. Immunizations are sometimes given, and occasionally treatment for common disorders such as dental caries and visual problems in low-income youngsters is provided. In the larger schools of the great cities, these services are often well developed, with full-time nurses on the premises, consulting psychologists, and periodic visits from physicians. Schools in rural districts, on the other hand, seldom have strong health programs. The isolated one-room country school house, of course, has handicaps in many spheres, but even in the larger schools of rural trade-centers the health programs tend to be weak. Instead of full-time school nurses, public health nurses from the health department, with many other duties, must cover the schools as well. Physicians are usually in too short supply to permit regular examinations of the children for detection of physical or mental defects.

Industrial establishments have also long provided special health protection, services, and safety-promotion programs for their workers. Large firms often have well-developed in-plant medical services, with full-time nurses, physicians, safety engineers, industrial hygienists, and others. Some of the earliest programs of prepaid medical care did, indeed, have their origins in isolated rural enterprises like mining, lumbering, and railroads.[41]

Most rural workers, however, do not have the benefit of good occupational health services. In smaller towns factories tend to have smaller work forces, and in-plant services are poorly developed. In the mines protective health and safety legislation is in effect, but the rate of serious injuries and fatal accidents is still high. Numerous small mines and lumbering operations have no organized medical or safety programs. In agriculture, of course, the majority of working people—whether self-employed farmers, tenants, or farm workers—are engaged in small enterprises without any occupational health programs. Even the large "agribusiness" farms or ranches seldom maintain the systematic health services found in urban factories with comparable numbers of employees. In such enterprises accident rates are often high, and a problem of serious concern in recent years has been the possible hazard to field workers from improper use of pesticides.[42]

The workmen's compensation laws on industrial injuries, which provide for disability cash payments and the costs of medical care, tend to be less comprehensive in the rural states. Self-employed farmers or tenants are not covered at all, and even agricultural employment is exempted from coverage under most state laws or left to the voluntary decision of the farm operator.[43]

Governmental medical care programs for special population groups under *federal* auspices are more equitable for rural people. Veterans with service-connected disabilities, wherever they may live, are entitled to first-class comprehensive medical care from the facilities of the U.S. Veterans Administration. Even for nonservice-connected conditions, veterans may get hospital care in any of 175 VA institutions if the verteran states that private care would be a financial hardship. Since this is usually true of the low-income veteran from a rural area, this federal program has particular value.[44] The same sort of rural benefit applies to the dependents of military personnel on active duty. Since 1956 these wives and children have been entitled to payment of most expenses for general medical care by the U.S. Department of Defense.

Among special diseases for which government assumes the major financial responsibility, mental disorder is the most important. Mental hospitals are nearly always a state government responsibility, and their quantity and quality in different states have been discussed previously. The modern approach to mental illness, however, is to attempt to treat emotional problems early so as to prevent the need for hospitalization. To facilitate this, a network of psychiatric clinics has been growing up around the nation, financed largely by grants from the federal and state governments.

The establishment and capacities of these mental health clinics are much weaker in the rural states. Psychiatrists are very heavily concentrated in the largest metropolitan centers (New York, Chicago, Los Angeles, etc.), and leadership in the small towns is usually lacking. Rural Arkansas, for example, has only four such psychiatric clinics, while urbanized Colorado with almost exactly the same state population (1,969,000) has twenty-eight of them. Urban Connecticut has fifty such clinics, while rural Iowa with just a slightly smaller population (2,760,000) has only twenty-two.[45] Perhaps the prevalence of mental disease is lower among more rural populations, but it is just as likely that the recognition of these problems is obscured by the inaccessibility of resources for their diagnosis and treatment.

Crippling conditions in children is another category of disorder that government has tackled. The U.S. Children's Bureau in the Department of Health, Education and Welfare gives grants to the states to help pay for the costs of medical care of children identified as "crippled" and financially eligible for this aid. These definitions are flexible, and the rural states actually derive relatively greater benefits from this program than the urban. In 1964 the crippled children's program served 5.1 children per 1000 persons under 21 years of age in the nation. Among the twenty most urban states, this average rate was exceeded in eight, while among the twenty most rural states it was exceeded in seventeen.[46] This special advantage for rural populations is not accidental, but has been deliberately written into the federal grant formula, which favors areas of greater poverty.

Disabled adults who are employable may be helped to get corrective medical care, as well as job training, by the federal grant-in-aid program of the Vocational Rehabilitation Administration (VRA). Eligibility, both medical and financial, is also flexible in this program, so that states with lower per capita incomes and fewer private resources tend to take greater advantage of it. Nationally the vocational rehabilitation program helped fifty-one persons per 100,000 in 1961—not a very large proportion. Among the twenty most rural states, however, this rate was exceeded in twelve, while in the twenty most urban states it was exceeded only in five. The greatest impact of the VRA program was in West Virginia (188 cases per 100,000) Georgia (152 cases), and Arkansas (138 cases), while the smallest relative impact was in California (16 cases per 100,000), Ohio (21 cases), and New Jersey (28 cases).[47]

Modern rehabilitation of disabled persons requires a combination of skills in physical medicine, surgery, vocational training, job counseling and placement, social casework, and other disciplines. Rehabilitation centers that offer these varied skills under one roof are not plentiful (there are only about 150 of them in the United States), and they are, of course, located in the larger cities. The governmental programs for children and adults just described usually arrange transportation of patients to these centers, not only covering travel costs, but also making the various professional and administrative liaisons required. Low-income rural people who are reached by these programs, therefore, may be greatly benefited, but those who must rely on their own private resources can seldom profit from the comprehensive rehabilitation centers in the metropolitan cities.

Voluntary health agencies

Complementing and often antedating governmental health programs are a great diversity of voluntary agencies with specific objectives for health service. Voluntary health insurance plans have been discussed, as have been the health activities of private industry; by contrast, the "voluntary health agency" does not have an earmarked population to cover. It is typically supported by charitable donations, and the benefits go to various and sundry persons in need of them.

There are thousands of voluntary health agencies in the United States, the best known of which conduct campaigns on specific diseases such as cancer, blindness, or cerebral palsy. Typically they devote their funds to a combination of support for scientific research, education of the health professions, and direct service to patients. The large voluntary organizations consist of a network of local chapters, state offices, and national headquarters that match governmental hierarchies in their complexity. In addition, there are many voluntary health agencies with purely local roots, directing their efforts to the solution of some unique local problem. It has been estimated that no less than 100,000 local voluntary units of both types are operating in the United States for various purposes.[48] Although the programs of these agencies do not compare in magnitude with those of government, and there is evidence of much waste because of fragmentation and high administrative overhead, nevertheless, they do help meet certain health needs not served by government, and they often pioneer new ideas.

As for other organized social efforts, however, the impact of the voluntary health agencies is typically lower in the rural areas. The sources of private charity are much greater in the cities, and health activities are largely carried out in the communities where the money is raised. Data form the American Heart Association, the voluntary health agency tackling the nations top cause of death, reflect the general tendency. This agency has chapters in every state, and it spends money in every state. In the fiscal year ending June 30, 1966, chapters spent over $21,000,000 or slightly over 10 cents per capita for the national population. This average of 10 cents, however, was exceeded in eight of the ten most urban states but in only two of the ten most rural states.[49] A similar computation of 1966 expenditures by the American Cancer Society showed outlays of over 20 cents per capita in thirteen out of the twenty-five most urban states, compared with only four out of the twenty-five most rural states.[50] Comparable relationships would undoubtedly be found for most of the other disease-specific voluntary agencies.

Some of the most important voluntary health agencies are virtually restricted to the large cities. Visiting nurse associations give bedside care to patients at home—usually the chronically ill of low income—but seldom do they serve rural populations. One striking exception is the Frontier Nursing Service of Kentucky, a philanthropically initiated program in which nurses go by jeep or horseback to serve isolated families in the backwoods. There are also some church missions providing small hospitals and general medical care for impoverished rural populations in New Mexico, Tennessee, and elsewhere. Other large agencies with national networks, however, such as Alcoholics Anonymous, the Salvation Army, or the Planned Parenthood Association, are essentially confined to the cities.

This is not to suggest that small towns and villages lack community spirit for health purposes. Women's home demonstration clubs, parent-teacher associations, church auxiliaries, and other such groups are numerous and active, and their programs may include some concern for issues like improved nutrition or safety on the school grounds. The purposes of such rurally based organizations, however, are mainly educational, and they have little direct impact on the medical needs of the rural poor.

Attracting physicians and others to rural areas

The previous pages have summarized the principal organized programs that help to meet the health needs of populations. Most of these programs are nationwide, with differential impacts on rural, compared with urban, people; some are specifically oriented to rural districts and to the poor within them. Underlying all these programs, however, is a need for health personnel and medical facilities to actually render the needed services. As we noted at the outset, these resources are in leaner supply and nearly always of poorer quality in the rural than in the urban areas. We must now examine, therefore, certain other general movements that are designed mainly to improve these basic human and material resources in rural areas.

Efforts to improve the rural supply of physicians have taken many forms. Basic is the output of physicians by the medical schools, since the overall national production of physicians naturally influences the number that will settle in rural areas. The net output of physicians by medical schools throughout the nation, however, has barely kept up with the growth of population over the last 30 years.[51] Indeed, were it not for the inflow of medical graduates of foreign medical schools in recent years, the net ratio would have markedly declined. Nevertheless, since the end of World War II there has been an increase from seventy-seven to eighty-eight medical schools in the United States—nearly all of the new ones being established by state governments. As of late 1966, moreover, sixteen more medical schools were in the process of development.[52] Enrollments in the existing schools have also been increased, although only slightly.

The principal growth of new medical schools in the last 20 years has been in the more rural states, like Kentucky, West Virginia, and New Mexico. These state-sponsored schools give preference to admission of native sons who, it may be expected, are more likely to settle in their home territory. Furthermore, an internship or residency at a university medical center often leads a young physician to start practice nearby, even if he or she comes originally from another state. Thus the establishment of new medical schools and teaching hospitals in the principal cities of rural regions is an important force for improving the supply of rural physicians in the long run. Federal grants to the universities for medical research, and more recently for medical school facility construction, have helped to foster this development.

Another approach to the problem of attracting physicians to rural areas has been the construction of modern office facilities. For many years small towns have taken it upon themselves to offer physicians rent-free office quarters or even low-cost homes to induce them to come.[53] In 1953 the Tennessee State Medical Association set up a "medical foundation" devoted to helping rural communities attract young physicians through advice on building private clinics and other means.[54] Since 1959 the Sears Roebuck Foundation has put money in back of this idea and conducted a systematic program of assisting small towns to build efficient private medical clinics, with capital loans and architectural plans. In 1966 twenty towns were so aided.[55] The American Medical Association has collaborated in this program, offering an "information service" to new medical graduates on towns and villages lacking a physician; since 1948 the AMA has held a series of "National Conferences on Rural Health," publicizing this and other approaches to the problem. In early 1967 Senator Tydings introduced in the U.S. Congress a "Rural Community Medical Clinic Loan Act," which would put the Sears Roebuck idea on a firm governmental basis; it would provide $10,000,000 in loans to rural communities of 500 to 5000 population for constructing clinic buildings to accomodate two or more private physicians. Amendments to the Health Professions' Educational Assistance Act in 1966, moreover, authorized forgiveness of educational loans up to 100% for physicians, dentists, and optometrists who set up practice in low-income rural areas.

Other steps have been taken by state governments to induce settlement of young physicians in rural localities. During and after World War II, several southern states enacted statutes to provide full fellowship support for medical students who, on completion of training, would set up practice in a rural community. The fellowships were given initially as loans, but the debts for up to 4 years of medical schooling were cancelled for each year that the young physician practiced in a community certified as "rural" by the state agency. This type of program is still operating in Kentucky, Virginia, North Carolina, and other states. In Virginia and Kentucky the State Department of Health administers the program, while in North Carolina it is a separate governmental "North Carolina Medical Care Commission."[56] The latter state also subsidizes the education of dentists and optometrists for rural practice, and the programs in the the several states differ in various details. Virginia's State Health Commissioner, however, comments: "It is hard to evaluate the effectiveness of the program. Certainly it has not been a great boon to (medical) practice in the rural areas; on the other hand, it has helped fill a monetary need for these students."[57]

Medical and surgical specialists are particularly lacking in rural areas, since, more than general practitioners, their successful practice requires the population concentration of the larger cities. For this reason the pattern of group medical practice, which can bring together a team of specialists and general physicians in a viable professional enterprise has great potentialities for betterment of rural medical care. It is encouraging, therefore, that group medical practice has been increasing significantly in rural counties, even though it is still a minority phenomenon.

In 1959 physicians engaged in multispeciality group practice (as distinguished from single specialty clusters) in the United States constituted a ratio of 5.8 per 100,000 civilian population.[58] While this is only a small percentage of the 132 physicians per 100,000 in the nation, it represented a marked increase from the level of 2.2 physicians per 100,000 in group practice in 1946. The ratio is decidedly higher, moreover, in the isolated rural counties where, in 1959, it was 8.2 such physicians per 100,000 compared with 5.0 in the metropolitan counties. As a proportion of total physicians in private practice, furthermore, the rural predominance of group practice is more striking, as shown by the following figures for 1959:

Type of county	Percentage of total private physicians in group practice
Metropolitan	4.6
Adjacent	8.0
Isolated	12.6

Probably more basic than these several strategies for attracting physicians to rural areas has been the construction and improvement of small-town hospitals, discussed earlier, and the extension of health insurance. Adequate facilities for medical practice and assurance of a satisfactory income are fundamental, although they cannot necessarily compensate for the cultural handicaps of small-town, as compared with large-city life. Between 1949 and

1959, however, the net effect of all the forces at play produced a slight decrease in the ratio of physicians in the metropolitan and adjacent counties (135.9 down to 132.6 per 100,000 population) and a slight increase in the ratio within the isolated counties (73.7 up to 74.7 per 100,000). As noted earlier, well-to-do country dwellers can readily travel to a distant city for medical care, but an improved physician supply within rural counties has special importance for the rural poor.

Attracting nurses and other types of allied personnel to rural districts is more directly dependent on organized measures, like hospital construction or health department enlargement, than is improvement of the physician supply. Paramedical personnel, more than physicians and dentists, are mainly employed in organized health agencies. Yet it is likely that the overall problem of rural health personnel will be most effectively solved within a framework of general improvement in the social and economic setting of rural community life.

Regionalization and comprehensive planning

The handicaps of rural ecology for the delivery of scientific medical service have led everywhere in the world to plans for greater use of transportation. Rural patients can be transported to an urban facility when necessary, or urban specialists can travel to the hinterland. Moreover, the entire level of technical performance in rural hospitals can be elevated by continuous professional and administrative ties to better developed urban institutions. Rural populations, in other words, can be served not only by the facilities in the country, but by a network of both rural and urban facilities covering large geographic regions.

This concept of hospital regionalization has had extensive discussion in the United States, although its actual accomplishments have so far been spotty. In 1936 a private foundation set out to improve the quality of medical care for the rural people of Maine, through organization of a system of professional connections between hospitals in the small towns of that state and a large medical center in Boston.[59] A somewhat similar network was organized in 1945 in the cluster of rural counties around Rochester, New York.[60] The principal impact of these programs has been to enrich the education of physicians, nurses, technicians, dieticians, and other personnel in rural hospitals, so as to improve their performance. Consultation services have gone from the center peripherally, but transfer of patients from the peripheral units to the center has occurred only occasionally. Upgrading the quality of small-town hospitals may be expected to benefit the poorer rural people particularly, since they are least likely to travel to a distant city for medical care.

The regionalization idea was emphasized along another dimension, with the enactment of the National Hospital Survey and Construction (Hill-Burton) Act of 1946. The basic purpose of this law was to promote construction of hospitals in areas of bed deficiency, and, as noted earlier in this report a remarkable equalization among the states was accomplished. Between 1948 and 1965 the population of the United States increased by 37%, while the general hospital bed supply increased by 70%. The relative bed increases were greater, moreover, in the more rural states. Among the twenty-five most urban states, fourteen enjoyed an increase in their bed-population ratios over this span of years, while among the twenty-five most rural states twenty benefitted by such an increase.[61] Not all this improvement can be attributed to the Hill-Burton Act, but the advantages for low-income states written into the federal granting formula suggest that in rural districts the improvement in hospital bed supply has been largely a result of the stimulus of this subsidy program. Between 1947 and 1966 nearly two-thirds of the $1,900,000,000 federal subsidy for general hospital construction went to communities of under 50,000 population.

Aside from their influence on quantitative improvement in hospital bed supplies, the state "master plans" required under the Hill-Burton Act affected the technical content of hospital design. On the one hand, minimum standards were set for laboratories, infant nurseries, outpatient departments, and other basic features found in all hospitals. On the other hand, excessively elaborate equipment was not allowed in rural facilities, so that complex cases would be referred to an urban center instead of being improperly handled locally. Furthermore, the Hill-Burton Act subsidized also the construction of "public health centers"—mainly to house local health departments—which helped to strengthen preventive and case-finding health services in low-income rural districts. Between 1948 and 1965 there were 726 primary public health centers and 328 auxiliary health centers constructed throughout the nation, the great majority under the stimulus of the Hill-Burton program.

With respect to hospital operations or the professional relationships among personnel in regional networks of facilities, the achievements of the last 20 years have not been so impressive. Bricks and mortar may be necessary to lay the foundations for regionalization, but they are obviously not enough to induce cooperative behavior among the component units in a geographic "system." One such theoretical system in northern Michigan, developed with the assistance of the Hill-Burton program and the Kellogg Foundation, was intensively studied over a 5-year period (1954 to 1959). Two small rural hospitals of nineteen and eighteen beds respectively were affiliated by a "regionalization agreement" with a 160-bed urban hospital forty miles away, and another small ten-bed rural hospital was affiliated with a 226-bed hospital twenty-five miles away. Various exchanges were to be developed in the way of consultation services, transfer of patients, professional education, joint purchasing of supplies, etc. In practice, however, very little of this was carried out, and the investigators concluded: "In essence regionalization, with its signed agreements, remained, on the whole, a paper achievement."[62]

Another regionalization effort, confined to the field of postgraduate medical education, was launched in the suburban and semirural districts encompassed in a seventy-five–mile radius around New York City. Fifteen small community hospitals were affiliated with the medical center of the New York University College of Medicine for a systematic program of continuing education through lectures and clinical case conferences offered by visiting professors. Local attendance, however, gradually diminished, interpersonal frictions developed, and after 17 years (1945 to 1962) the program was terminated.[63] Other medical schools, which have launched similar educational programs, have not reported great success, and they may well be less candid than New York University in admitting failures.

Since about 1957 the hospital regionalization idea has come to have an additional meaning other than that just discussed. Instead of providing a framework for bringing sound medical care to rural residents of large geographic areas, it has been applied to the developmental problems of hospitals within metropolitan centers. In the great cities there are plenty of fiscal and administrative problems in the planning of hospital construction; the unfettered building of new hospitals—without considering the optimal use of the existing facilities—has led to wasteful inefficiencies. To cope with this, community leaders in Chicago, Pittsburgh, and other large cities organized "voluntary hospital councils," representing philanthropic sources (usually local industrialists) as well as the hospitals themselves.[64] Through various indirect financial and moral pressures, these councils have attempted to influence the pattern of new hospital construction, or the renovation of existing facilities. They have also promoted certain joint administrative and professional practices (such as recruitment or in-service training of personnel) among the hospitals within the city.[65] By 1966 there were about fifty of these metropolitan councils in the nation, many of which had been stimulated and sustained by special federal grants authorized under the 1960 Hill-Harris amendments to the Hill-Burton Act. While doubtless helping to optimize the nation's net investment in hospital construction, these metropolitan councils have done little to meet the special problems of rural populations, and especially of the rural poor.

It is not surprising, therefore, that in 1965 a very different approach to the problem of upgrading rural medical care through regionalization was taken by the federal government. Focusing on the nation's three leading causes of death—heart disease, cancer, and stroke—Congress enacted amendments to the Public Health Service Act to provide grants-in-aid for "regional medical programs . . . for research, training, diagnosis, and treatment relating to heart disease, cancer, or stroke." The intent is to promote much stronger ties than those presently existing between the great urban medical centers and the smaller hospitals or other health facilities in far-flung rural regions.[66] As in the earlier regionalization programs, the greatest emphasis seems to be placed on postgraduate education and consultation to local physicians in the smaller hospitals. It remains to be seen whether the potentialities of this program for improving the quality of medical service to the rural poor will be realized, at least with respect to the major killing diseases.

Finally, a still more far-reaching step has recently been taken by the federal government toward potential improvement of rural health service, by way of both geographic and functional planning. Public Law 89-749, enacted in 1966, provides for federal grants to the states for "comprehensive health planning" of all health services, facilities, and manpower.[67] This is a wider definition of health planning authority than had so far been made by government in the United States, with clear intent to encompass both governmental and private activities and financial support for the planning efforts. The new law calls for coordination of programs supported by local and state as well as federal funds; it sets as a goal the achievement of high quality health service, both preventive and curative, for everyone. Planning, of course, is only a first step toward remedial action. If this step is taken in each state, the groundwork can be laid to increase the quantity of medical resources, to elevate their quality, and to coordinate their impact on the health needs of all rural people.*

Problems that must be solved

This report has examined the health needs and services of the rural poor, the organized programs operating to cope with the problems, and the deficiencies of the current situation. What can be done to improve the health of low-income rural people and to reduce the gap between medical science and its application? What specific problems must be solved?

In the account of past and current programs of health service, clues to future answers are implicit. The essentials are easy enough to state as ultimate goals:

1. The resources both in personnel and facilities for sound health service must be made available
2. Economic support for these services to all rural people, year in and year out, must be assured
3. The quality of health service must be maintained through reasonable measures of social organization

The attainment of these broad goals is not so easy. Certainly they could not be reached within the boundaries of life of the rural poor, nor of the rural population generally. Action would be necessary at the national level, as well as within rural states and communities. Moreover, changes would be necessary in the larger social and economic scene, as well as within the sphere of the health services.

Thus approaches to the solution of the health problems of the rural poor

---

*In 1976 both the Regional Medical Program and the Comprehensive Health Planning Act were replaced by the National Health Planning and Resources Development Act (see Chapter 1).

may be suggested at three levels: (1) the total rural economy, (2) the national health scene, and (3) the local rural health field.

At the level of the total rural economy, it is obvious that many social improvements are essential to attainment of better health service. Elevation of rural family incomes is basic. Based on firmer agricultural and industrial foundations, improved housing would be necessary, whether in the small town or village or out in the open country. Better education is needed in elementary and high schools; all rural youth who can profit from it should be free to undertake higher education. While transportation has greatly improved, still more development is needed to connect isolated villages with the main cities. Higher incomes and better education would lay the groundwork for further measures of health protection, such as sound nutrition and hygienic behavior. Segregation of minorities and racial discrimination in all its forms must be eliminated.

At the second level, the national health scene, several actions are necessary to achieve better health services for the rural poor. It is naive to expect the problems to be solved within the confines of rural communities. This would be true even if the total rural economy were highly advanced, but it is all the more so in the light of rural economic inequities that prevail and may be realistically expected to continue for some years. At the national level, health actions are needed in four main spheres.

Health manpower must be produced in much greater numbers if the needs of rural and urban people are to be met. So long as the total supply is not adequate, redistribution of health personnel between city and country will help very little; the rural locations will remain at the bottom of the national barrel. Increased production of physicians, dentists, nurses, technicians, and other health personnel will require further support from national and state governments. At the same time, new types of health workers, such as technical aides and assistants with skills appropriate to modern medical teamwork, should be explored; the alternative is nostalgic retention of the patterns of horse-and-buggy solo medical practice.

Second, the material foundations of medical service must be further strengthened through national action. Hospitals and health centers must be built wherever they are needed, with national economic assistance for construction as well as equipment.

Third, and extremely important, an economic arrangement must be made to pay for all the medical care that anyone needs. This complex requirement has had hundreds of piecemeal solutions in America. The achievements of voluntary health insurance have been reviewed in the pages above, as well as the great step forward of the Medicare law for the aged. Rural people, however, and especially the rural poor, are not well covered by voluntary insurance; even the fraction of the rural poor who are insured do not have comprehensive medical benefits. Continued efforts may enroll more of them in voluntary plans, but the soundest solution would undoubtedly be extension of the social insurance principle of Medicare to cover all age groups. Benefits should likewise be broadened to include physician's care in the office and home, as well as hospital service, dental care, prescribed drugs, and miscellaneous paramedical services.

If national comprehensive health insurance is enacted, many of the categorical programs discussed earlier would no longer be needed. The welfare medical services, with all their complex administrative features, are an awkward adjustment to the lack of national insurance; likewise for the Veterans Administration program, the crippled children's services, the workmen's compensation medical entitlements, and all the other fragmented health programs. Special grants for migrant families and an independent program for reservation Indians would be obviated if everyone were protected by national health insurance. All these rural people would be encompassed in the main economic stream of medical care. If special health centers were needed to reach isolated families, they would be financed by the national health insurance fund. For low-income persons who could not pay social insurance contributions, welfare agencies would pay the necessary premiums.

The fourth type of action needed at the national level concerns the multifarious problems of quality maintenance. Drug production, for example, obviously requires national controls, since the pharmaceutical industry is nationwide. Standards for medical specialty certification are now national, though voluntary, and the same is true of hospital accreditation. Similar promulgation and enforcement of national quality standards are needed in all other sectors of health service, including even basic professional licensure, which can no longer be scientifically justified on a state-by-state basis. Rural communities, more than urban, can benefit from the discipline of such national standards.

At the third level, the local rural health field, further actions are necessary. Even within the states and the rural communities, effective steps need some partial assistance from higher political levels, but distinct local measures are still feasible along five lines.

Rural public health agencies in counties or larger multicounty districts need great strengthening. Their role should not only be to promote health education, environmental sanitation, and other preventive services, but also to coordinate all the preventive and curative services in the area. It is the local health department that should set up convenient health centers to serve seasonal agricultural workers, psychiatric clinics, cancer detection units, or rehabilitation centers. Likewise, the health department should oversee the local hospitals and nursing homes with respect to quality standards. National health insurance may pay most of the operating costs, but leadership is still necessary to organize the local technical resources.

Second, rural hospitals can be greatly improved in their internal organization. The economic support and quality standards proposed above will contribute to this, but local initiative by citizen boards of directors is still necessary. New patterns like that of the Hunterdon Medical Center, with a stable staff of hospital-based specialists supplemented by visiting general practitioners, should be launched in more rural communities.[68]

Third, medical personnel should be attracted to rural communities much more systematically than they are now. The training of medical and dental students is already largely at social expense; even if they pay their own tuition, the latter covers only a small fraction of educational costs. It would be reasonable, therefore, to expect all new graduates to serve for a period in rural areas of need, as is widely required in other nations. Combined with the economic support of national health insurance, the provision of good hospitals and health centers, and a general increase in medical manpower, this policy could assure parity of physicians to serve rural people.

Fourth, there is the large task of breathing real life into the concept of health care regionalization. The planning of hospital construction along regional lines has made progress, but functional ties among the facilities in geographic regions are hardly developed. Implementation of the newly authorized regional medical programs for heart disease, cancer, and stroke requires far more imaginative action than has been shown in current projects, with their overwhelming attention devoted to postgraduate medical courses. Comprehensive health service planning, called for by further new legislation, must find ways to bring the benefits of urban medical science to the humblest village dweller.

Fifth, there remains the challenge of local voluntary action. Health service cooperatives can organize group practice clinics, which bring specialty services to the countryside on an efficient and economical basis. Rural hospitals and health centers can always benefit from volunteer support. New ideas in better health care can be pioneered by local voluntary groups, long before government agencies at any level are able to act.

These five forms of health action at the local rural level, along with the major steps recommended at the national level, are no small challenge. They would be costly in effort and dollars, though easily within our economic capacity. Their benefits must be measured in both material and human values. The effects of improved health on economic productivity require no argument. But the value of a pain that is soothed, a wound that is dressed, a life that is saved goes beyond the happiness of the individual. The opportunity to receive the benefits of medical science and enjoy good health has become a basic human right. It has been articulated from the podium of the United Nations and the doorstep of the country store.[69] Without this opportunity, families and communities can become demoralized and lose the will to act effectively in other spheres.[70] With health services assured, the millions of poor people in rural America can be encouraged to tackle more energetically the many other social and economic problems they face. Their lives can attain the quality of which this nation is capable.

References

1. Stern, B. J.: Society and medical progress, Princeton, N.J., 1941, Princeton University Press, pp. 126-141.
2. Winslow, C.-E. A.: The cost of sickness and the price of health, Geneva, 1951, World Health Organization.
3. Mott, F. D., and Roemer, M. I.: Rural health and medical care, New York, 1948, McGraw-Hill Book Co., pp. 50-73.
4. Lerner, M., and Anderson, O. W.: Health progress in the United States 1900-60, Chicago, 1963, University of Chicago Press, pp. 105-113.
5. U.S. Public Health Service: Vital and health statistics: data from the National Health Survey: acute conditons, incidence and associated disability, United States, July, 1962-June, 1963, Washington, D.C., 1965, U.S. Government Printing Office.
6. U.S. Public Health Service: Vital and health statistics: age patterns in medical care, illness, and disability, United States, July, 1963-June, 1965, Washington, D.C., 1966, U.S. Government Printing Office.
7. U.S. Public Health Service: Vital and health statistics: disability days, United States, July, 1963- June, 1964, Washington, D. C., 1965, U.S. Government Printing Office.
8. U.S. Army, Office of the Surgeon General: Results of the examination of youths for military service 1965 (supplement to Health of the Army), vol. 21, July 1966, p. 15.
9. U.S. Public Health Service: Vital and health statistics: medical care, health status, and family income, United States, Washington, D.C., 1964, U.S. Government Printing Office.
10. U.S. Public Health Service: Health manpower source book, Sec. 18, Manpower in the 1960's, Washington, D.C., 1964, U.S. Government Printing Office, p. 25.
11. Greenhill, S., and Singh, H. J.: Comparison of the professional functions of rural and urban general practitioners, J. Med. Educ. **40**:856-861, September 1965.
12. U.S. Public Health Service: Health manpower source book, Sec. 19, Location of manpower in eight health occupations, 1962, Washington, D.C., 1962, U.S. Government Printing Office, p. 27.
13. U.S. Public Health Service: Health resources statistics: health manpower, 1965, PHS Pub. No. 1509, Washington, D.C., 1967, U.S. Government Printing Office.
14. U.S. Public Health Service: Health manpower source book, Sec. 2, Nursing personnel, Washington, D.C., 1966, U.S. Government Printing Office, p. 12.
15. Peterson, O. L., Andrews, L. P., Spain, R. S., and Greenberg, B. G.: Analytical study of North Carolina general practice 1953-54, J. Med. Educ. **31** (12, Part II):1-165, 1956.
16. Mott, F. D., and Roemer, M. I.:*op. cit,* pp. 217-244.
17. U.S. Public Health Service: Hill-Burton state plan data: hospital and medical facilities series: a national summary, Washington, D.C., 1965, U.S. Government Printing Office, pp. 42-45.
18. Based on statistics in American Hospital Association: guide issue, Hospitals, p. 430, August 1961.
19. *Ibid.*
20. U.S. Public Health Service: Nursing homes and related facilities—fact book, PHS Pub. No. 930-F-4, Washington, D.C., February 1963, U. S. Government Printing Office, pp. 10-13.
21. U.S. Public Health Service: Hill-Burton state plan data: hospital and medical facilities series: a national summary, Washington, D.C., 1965, U.S. Government Printing Office, pp. 57-60.
22. Hollingshead, A. B., and Redlich, F. C.: Social class and mental illness, New York, 1958, John Wiley and Sons, Inc.
23. American Nurses' Association: Facts about nursing, New York, 1966, American Nurses' Association, pp. 220-221.
24. U.S. Public Health Service: Vital and health statistics: age patterns in medical care, illness, and disability, United States, July, 1963-June, 1965, Washington, D.C., 1966, U.S. Government Printing Office.
25. U.S. Public Health Service: Directory of local health units 1964, Washington, D.C., 1965, U.S. Government Printing Office, p. 74.
26. U.S. Welfare Administration: Welfare in review: statistical supplement, 1966 edition, Washington, D.C., 1966, U.S. Government Printing Office, p. 39.
27. *Ibid.,* p. 13.

28. Anderson, O.W., and Feldman, J.J.: Family medical costs and voluntary health insurance: a nationwide survey, New York, 1956, McGraw-Hill Book Co. (Blakiston Division).

29. Health Insurance Institute: 1966 Source book of health insurance data, New York, 1967, The Institute, p. 5.

30. United Mine Workers of America, Welfare and Retirement Fund: Report for the year ending June 30, 1966, Washington, D.C., 1967, U.S. Government Printing Office.

31. Somers, H. M., and Somers, A. R.: Doctors, patients, and health insurance, Washington, D.C., 1961, The Brookings Institution, p. 272.

32. Reed, L. J.: The extent of health insurance coverage in the United States, U.S. Social Security Administration, Research Report No. 10, Washington, D.C., 1965, U.S. Government Printing Office, pp. 59-60.

33. U.S. Social Security Administration: Independent health insurance plans in the United States: 1965 survey, Research Report No. 17, Washington, D.C., 1966, U.S. Government Printing Office, pp. 44-45.

34. U.S. Social Security Administration: Data provided by L. Bernstein, March 29, 1967.

35. Based on data in Is the medicare program meeting the nation's need? Med. World News, pp. 68-78, April 14, 1967.

36. Mott, F. D., and Roemer, M. I.: *op. cit.,* pp. 389-431.

37. U.S. Senate Committee on Labor and Public Welfare: The migratory farm labor problem in the United States: 1965 report, Washington, D.C., 1965, U.S. Government Printing Office, pp. 6-10.

38. U.S. Senate Committee on Labor and Public Welfare: Interim report on the status of program activities under the migrant health act (submitted by the U.S. Public Health Service), Washington, D.C., 1964, U.S. Government Printing Office.

39. Wagner, C. J., and Rabeau, E. S.: Indian poverty and Indian health, Indicators, U.S. Dept. of Health, Education and Welfare, Washington, D.C., March 1964, U.S. Government Printing Office, pp. 24-54.

40. U. S. Department of Health, Education and Welfare: To improve medical care, Revised edition, Washington, D.C., April 1966, U.S. Government Printing Office, p. 49.

41. Williams, P.: The purchase of medical care through fixed periodic payment, New York, 1932, National Bureau of Economic Research.

42. Haller, H. L.: Pesticides: the challenge— how do we meet it? Am J. Public Health 54 (part II):37-41, January 1964.

43. Skolnik, A. M.: Twenty-five years of workmen's compensation statistics, Soc. Security Bull., pp. 3-26, October 1966.

44. Cohen, I. J.: The veterans administration medical care program. In DeGroot, L. J., editor: Medical care: social and organizational aspects, Springfield, Ill., 1966, Charles C Thomas, publisher.

45. U.S. Public Health Service: Outpatient psychiatric clinics, psychiatric day-night services, 1963 directory, PHS Pub. No. 1129, Washington, D.C., June 1964, U.S. Government Printing Office.

46. U.S. Welfare Administration: Welfare in review: statistical supplement for 1966, Washington, D.C., 1967, U.S. Government Printing Office, p. 41.

47. U.S. Department of Health, Education and Welfare: Health education and welfare trends, Washington, D.C., 1962, U.S. Government Printing Office, p. 151.

48. Hamlin, R.: Voluntary health and welfare agencies in the United States, New York, 1961, Schoolmaster's Press.

49. American Heart Association (New York Headquarters): Data provided by Castranova, S. J., April 17, 1967.

50. American Cancer Society (New York Headquarters): Data provided by Bullock, A., April 28, 1967.

51. Surgeon General's Consultant Group on Medical Education: Physicians for a growing America, Washington, D.C., 1959, U.S. Public Health Service.

52. Council on Medical Education and Hospitals: Undergraduate medical education: medical schools, J.A.M.A. **198**:851, November 21, 1966.

53. Roemer, M. I.: Approaches to the rural doctor shortage, Rural Sociology, **16**:137-147, June 1951.

54. Massie, W. A.: Medical services for rural areas: the Tennessee Medical Foundation, Cambridge, 1957, Harvard University Press.

55. M.D.'s obtained for rural areas: AMA News, February 27, 1967.

56. North Carolina Medical Care Commission: Educational loans for medical and related studies, Raleigh, N.C., 1967.

57. Virginia State Department of Health: Data provided by M. I. Shanholtz, April 3, 1967.

58. U.S. Public Health Service: Medical groups in the United States, 1959, PHS Pub. No.

1063, Washington, D.C., 1963, U.S. Government Printing Office, p. 25.

59. Smillie, W. G., and Curran, J. A.: The unmet needs in medical care of rural people. state of Maine, Bethel, Maine, 1957, Bingham Associates Fund.

60. Rosenfeld, L. S., Makover, H. B.: The Rochester Regional Hospital Council, Cambridge, 1956, Commonwealth Fund.

61. U.S. Public Health Service: Hill-Burton state plan data: hospital and medical facilities series: a national summary, Washington, D.C., 1965, U.S. Government Printing Office.

62. McNerney, W. J., and Riedel, D. C.: Regionalization and rural health care (an experiment in three communities), Ann Arbor, Mich., 1962, The University of Michigan Press, p. 156.

63. de la Chapelle, C. E., and Jensen, F.: A mission in action: the story of the Regional Hospital Plan of New York University, New York, 1964, New York University Press.

64. Myers, R. S.: Areawide planning for hospitals leads to good medical services, Mod. Hosp., p. 114, December 1961.

65. Sigmond, R.: Regional hospital planning under voluntary or governmental auspices, Hosp. Forum, June 1963.

66. Marston, R. Q., and Yordy, K.: A nation starts a program: regional medical programs, 1965-1966, J. Med. Educ. 42:17-27, January 1967.

67. Public Law 89-749: Comprehensive health planning and public health services amendments of 1966.

68. Trussell, R. E.: Hunterdon Medical Center: the story of one approach to rural medical care, Cambridge, 1956, Harvard University Press.

69. Brockington, F.: World health, London, 1958, Penguin Books, pp. 208-235.

70. Harrington, M.: The other America: poverty in the United States, New York, 1962, The Macmillan Co.

CHAPTER 5

Rural health care solutions attempted around the world

In virtually all countries rural populations suffer health service disadvantages, relative to urban populations. Even though many of the health problems caused by urban congestion would seem to be less severe in rural districts, the sociotechnical advantages of urban settlement have usually more than compensated for these handicaps. The rural areas almost everywhere have been "left behind" in the development of modern health services. Especially serious is the problem of maldistribution of physicians, hospitals, and other resources, and the resultant deficiencies in the rate of health services received by rural people.

To take a bird's-eye view of an enormously heterogeneous world, nine large topics are examined briefly, as they are seen in various countries, with the solutions attempted in diverse settings. These topics are: (1) the health problems of rural people, (2) organized actions to prevent disease, (3) efforts to attract or direct physicians to rural areas, (4) the expanding use of ancillary health personnel, (5) extension of rural hospitals and health centers (for ambulatory care), (6) improvement of transportation and communication, (7) the promotion and maintenance of health care quality, (8) extension of economic support for health services to rural people, and (9) the movement everywhere for greater planning and coordination of health services for rural and urban populations.

A brief review of actions that have been taken to cope with these problems in countries throughout the world was presented at a conference on "Rural and Appalachian Health" held in 1972. This was published as one chapter of a book reporting the proceedings of this conference: Nolan, R. L., and Schwartz, J. L., editors: *Rural and Appalachian Health*, Springfield, Ill., 1973, Charles C Thomas, Publisher, pp. 65-78.

Rural health problems

Deficiencies in health services among rural populations are found in every country of the world. In the poorest countries to the richest, in the most agricultural and underdeveloped nations to the most industrialized and highly developed, the rural population tends to receive a lower level of health service in relation to its needs than the urban population. This is found both by quantitative measures of services utilized and by estimates of the quality of those services.

Striking evidence for this has recently been produced by a national study in Colombia, South America, where a higher incidence of illness was found among rural people by household surveys (both interviews and medical examiniations) than among urban; yet there was a lower volume of ambulatory and hospital services received by rural people, even counting the ministrations of nonscientific healers. In the developing countires generally, village dwellers get a higher proportion of their limited volume of medical care from traditional healers than do city-dwellers; they also depend more heavily on self-prescribed drugs. In the United States the mortality among rural people is somewhat lower than among urban people, but the volume of sickness, especially chronic, is higher; the utilization of ambulatory medical and dental services and of hospitalization is distinctly lower.

To cope with these inequities, almost all countries have undertaken special efforts to compensate for the inherent handicaps of the rural environment. These efforts are nearly always put forth at the national level. It seems to be generally recognized that the solution of rural health care problems must be like the treatment of a systemic disease; the rural symptom is only a manifestation of a systemic disorder, and to alleviate or cure it, actions must be taken to modify the functioning of the total system.

For the sake of brevity, I should like to oversimplify a very diversified array of social actions to cope with rural health care problems, and consider them under eight categories. In practice, actions in each of these spheres are obviously interrelated to actions in the other spheres, and the overall effort is heavily influenced by the general sociopolitical design of the health service system. Yet it is interesting to observe how much commonality there is to certain types of health measures even among countries at different points on the political spectrum and at different stages of economic development.

Prevention of disease

The prevention of disease or promotion of health through environmental or mass population measures figures prominently in rural health improvement efforts everywhere. In the developing countries vector-borne diseases, such as malaria or schistosomiasis, are highly prevalent in rural populations and are the object of environmental control campaigns. Measures to control such diseases through filling in swamps, spraying houses with insecticides, eliminating snails from streams, etc. are usually launched by central governments, even when there is a local health agency available for personal health services. Improvements in rural water supplies and excreta disposal systems have been a very slow process, and in the developing countries have usually also depended on provision of equipment and technical aid from central ministries of health.

The most widespread preventive efforts in personal health service have been in the promotion of maternal and child health. The periodic examination of the expectant woman and the check-up of the small infant with immunizations, advice on proper feeding, and hygienic counseling are a staple of rural health programs in Latin America, Asia, and Africa, as much as in Europe and North America. In the developing world these examinations and advice are typically given by midwives and other auxiliary personnel, rarely by physicians. Moreover, in these countries the sharp distinction between prevention and treatment applied in the United States is seldom found in rural programs (though it persists in the larger cities); the sick infant is treated to the extent possible. A common program in rural health centers is the rehydration (through parenteral fluids) of infants dehydrated from gastrointestinal disease. The effectiveness of these MCH programs is reflected by the decline almost everywhere of rural infant mortality over the last 30 or 40 years, even though it generally remains higher than the urban mortality.

Reduced infant mortality has led in many countries of Asia and Africa and less so in Latin America to another form of prevention, family planning. With declines in death rates, population growth has accelerated. The large field of population control and family plannning cannot be discussed here, except to note that in India, Thailand, Ghana, and elsewhere, contraceptive programs have been incorporated in the rural MCH activities. Insertions of intrauterine devices and male sterilization procedures are done by physicians, but dispensing of pills and contraceptive instructions of other types are usually done by rural nurses or midwives. Chile, under its new Marxist government, seems to be the first Latin American country to incorporate family planning into its national health policy.

Getting physicians to rural areas

Concentrations of physicians in the large cities is a worldwide phenomenon. To some extent, of course, this is quite reasonable, insofar as cities must be centers for serving large regions with highly specialized care. But the resultant shortages of physicians in the small towns serving rural districts are often severe, and a variety of corrective actions have been taken.

Most basic has been the expansion everywhere of medical schools, in order to produce a greater national output of physicians. So long as the national supply is deficient, the rural areas with their general cultural handicaps will attract the fewest medical graduates. The most impressive increases in the total output of physicians have occurred in the Soviet Union and other socialist countries; Cuba, for example, has much more than made up for its massive exodus of physicians following the 1959 revolution, and now has over 7000 physicians for its 8,000,000 people—a ratio (about 1:1150) about equal to that of the Scandinavian countries a few years ago. Nearly all the Latin American countries have achieved improved ratios of physicians over the last 30 years, and the establishment of medical schools in the newly emancipated countries of Africa is accomplishing the same.

After production of physicians, of course, the task is to bring about their distribution in relation to population needs, and various methods have been used. Since about 1935 Mexico has made a period of "social service" in a rural village a condition for earning the medical degree; originally this was for 6 months, and now it is for 1 year. An increasing number of countries in Latin America and Asia are doing likewise. Indonesia and Turkey have such requirements; Iran achieves this end through a period of service in the Rural Health Corps, as a form of military obligation. Malaysia has recently instituted a 2-year rural service requirement, in connection with the output of the first graduating class from its own medical school (formerly its physicians had to be trained abroad). The Soviet Union requires 3 years of service by new medical graduates in a rural health center.

Several states in our country have had "rural medical fellowship" programs since the 1940's, including Virginia and North Carolina. The new graduate serves 1 year in a rural area of need for each medical school year in which he or she has received fellowship support. The recently passed Emergency Health Personnel Act of 1970 is the first federal approach to the problem, using military obligations as the device for getting physicians to rural areas; appropriations for implementation of this law are still being awaited.

The more difficult task is to hold physicians in rural areas after an initial period. The experience of the mandatory rural service programs, both in the United States and elsewhere, is that when the statutory obligation is fulfilled the young physician usually leaves for a city. In the Soviet Union, this tendency is countered by payment of higher salaries for a rural than for a comparable urban position. Similar salary differentials for rural work have recently been introduced in Mexico.

Assuring a satisfactory income is, of course, basic to solution of the rural physician problem. Even though earnings are obviously not the whole story, we know that in the United States physician incomes in the villages are lower than those in all cities except the multimillion population metropolises. Various schemes have been used to guarantee rural incomes. In the rural municipalities of the Canadian prairie provinces, salaries have been paid to general practitioners by local government since 1917. The Highlands and Islands Scheme of northern Scotland pays salaries to physicians who could not hope to make an adequate income from the sparse population in this region. New Zealand has similar arrangements in isolated localities, administered by the national Ministry of Health. Coal-mining communities in West Virginia and other Appalachian states have long supported physicians through salaries paid from local employer-employee prepayment plans. The basic issue of adequate income support for physicians and others in rural health service is, of course, tied up with the general problem of economic support, which will be explored below.

Other conditions besides income designed to keep physicians in rural places include provision of housing. Many American towns offer an attractive house at very low rental as an inducement. In the developing countries, government-financed housing is a standard feature of rural assignments for the physician, along with other health personnel. Office quarters at low rentals have also been offered to physicians by small towns in Canada and the United States; many of these are small health centers built with the assistance of the Sears Roebuck Foundation. The provision of modern rural hospitals, of course, is also an attraction for physicians—a basic premise in back of the Hill-Burton hospital construction program in this country.

In Great Britain rural settlement of physicians is encouraged by a national policy of designating certain areas as "over-doctored"; in these areas, typically metropolitan, new physicians are not permitted to settle—at least not under the financial support of the National Health Service. As a result, the physicians going elsewhere will sometimes be channeled to rural communities. There was a somewhat similar policy in West Germany, where the local sickness funds with heavy medical participation used to prohibit new physicians from settling, thereby compelling them to settle in areas of greater need; unfortunately for rural areas, a recent German court decision invalidated this policy in the interest of "free trade" for the medical profession. Tunisia, on the other hand, is a country that has banned new physicians from settling in the busy national capital, Tunis, thereby diverting them to other towns. All similar policies obviously require national health planning and the exercise of considerable control over the flow of funds to pay for medical care.

Ancillary health manpower

The use of personnel other than physicians to meet health needs has been more extensively applied in rural areas than in cities throughout the world. The well-known "feldsher" of Czarist Russia was originally a rural medical replacement for the physician. After the revolution, with the great increase in physician output, there was an intention to eliminate this type of health worker as substandard, but ultimately the feldsher was kept. He or she now works in both rural and urban areas as a general medical auxiliary, with wider responsibilities than the nurse; in rural posts the feldsher serves villages of a few hundred people, too few to warrant a full-time physician. An important feature of the Soviet manpower model is the freedom of feldshers or nurses to undertake further studies and become physicians; this is one of the reasons that so many Soviet physicians are women.

Many countries have trained special classes of middle-level health personnel for rural service. Ethiopia has its famous Public Health Training College at Gondar, where "health officers" are trained for both curative and preventive work in rural health centers; their curriculum requires 3 years of study after high school, followed by 1 year of supervised field work. Community nurses and sanitarians are similarly trained in relatively short periods. Venezuela has its rural program of so-called simplified medicine, staffed by auxiliary nurses and male medical assistants. In Ceylon rural posts are staffed by dispensers of common remedies, who are still quaintly called "apothecaries." In Malaysia the old British term of "hospital assistant" is applied to male health personnel who give the curative service in rural health centers, while nurses and nursing assistants give the preventive service. Throughout Africa the "dresser," a male auxiliary with very little formal schooling, is the commonest source of medical care, outside of primitive healers, for most of the rural population.

Most of the world's infants are undoubtedly delivered by midwives, who have learned their skills simply from observation and experience. Throughout Asia and Africa, and less so in Latin America, young village women with grade-school education have been given formal training of 1 or 2 years to serve as "government midwives." The task everywhere is to win over the rural people to use these trained midwives, rather than the untrained ones with whom they are usually more familiar. The trained midwife, of course, is by no means limited to rural areas of underdeveloped countries. She is the attendant at most childbirths in Great Britain and Holland, where the infant and maternal mortality records are, incidentally, better than in the United States.

The hundreds of millions of people in rural China have long depended on herbalists and acupuncturists for their medical care. Under the current Communist government, thousands of young peasants have been trained to offer immunizations, first aid for injuries, scientific drugs for common diseases, and education about personal hygiene. These "barefoot doctors," as they are called, are now the mainstays of rural health care in the People's Republic, working as part of a network of both Western and traditional medicine in each province.

Rural hospitals and health centers

Insofar as local wealth has financed hospital construction, rural populations have always been left behind. This has been true in the wealthy United States no less than in India or Brazil. It took the Hill-Burton Act in our country, with its strong priorities for rural states and the rural regions within every state, to improve the relative hospital bed supply for rural people. Over the last 25 years since this program was started, bed supply has been quite well equalized between rural and urban areas; in fact, the dynamics of patient flow today are such that the greater pressures of bed shortage are being felt in the city hospitals that are serving both urban and rural people.

Hospital construction in the main provincial towns serving rural districts is a standard objective in the ministry of health plans in countries of Latin America, Asia, and Africa. While urban hospitals are often built by voluntary bodies or purely private groups, rural district hospitals nearly always depend on central government; the chief exception are the hospitals, usually small, established by foreign religious missions. Throughout Latin America, and also in Iran and Turkey, social security agencies, separate from health ministries, have built many large well-equipped hospitals; these are limited, however, to their beneficiaries who are nearly always industrial or commercial workers in the main cities.

The rural district hospital outside of Western Europe and North America typically has much responsibility for ambulatory care. Its outpatient department provides the specialty care for the whole district, since private specialists are nonexistent in these areas. In Great Britain all hospitals come under the control of Regional Hospital Boards, which attempt to coordinate the response to needs both in cities and in the rural sections around them. Sweden also has a regionalization scheme, under which graded responsibilities are assigned to rural, district, and provincial hospitals. The hospital in Chile is administratively responsible for all official health services, ambulatory and environmental, in its catchment area. This is the pattern also in the Soviet Union.

Probably more important on a world scale than the rural hospital is the rural health center, a facility for ambulatory service, curative and preventive. There are different intensities of staffing. In Mexico, for example, there are the type A health centers, which are staffed by several physicians with specialty qualifications and located in the main provincial towns; the type B centers are staffed by one general medical practitioner aided by nurses and other auxiliaries; and type C centers in small villages are staffed only by auxiliary personnel and visited occasionally by a supervising physician. Malaysia and Thailand have their "main health centers," staffed by one physician and several nurses and auxiliaries, and "subcenters" staffed only by auxiliary personnel. In sub-Sahara Africa, the health centers are usually staffed only by dressers and assistant nurses, with physicians found only at district hospitals. Sometimes a health center will contain a few beds for some maternity cases or emergencies, pending referrral to a hospital. The smallest rural facilities are sometimes called rural posts or stations, where a single health auxiliary, with a small supply of government-supplied drugs, lives in a village.

Health centers, staffed by a general practitioner and a pediatrican, along with nurses and others, are the standard facility for ambulatory care in the rural areas of the socialist countries of Eastern Europe. In the main cities, where specialists are found, the ambulatory units are considered polyclinics, although generalists also work in them. It is interesting to note theat Great Britain, after great initial resistance to the idea by general practitioners, is now rapidly developing health centers for housing family physicians along with public health nurses and social workers. The general practitioner sees the patients on his or her panel and is paid by capitation; he or she is usually not a salaried employee. Such health centers are now being built by local health authorities both in large English and Scottish cities and in small towns. A similar movement is starting in New Zealand, even though the general practitioners under this country's national health service are paid by fee-for-service.

On every continent the concept of an orderly network of facilities is developing, with health centers operating as satellites of hospitals. Patients are sent from the health center to the hospital for diagnostic workups and treatment; after hospital discharge, the patient is referred back to the health center for follow-up care. In the Soviet Union a regular policy of exchange of positions is carried out between health centers and hospitals for 1 or 2 months per year, so that the physician in each setting can learn about the problems in the other setting. In the United States the "neighborhood health centers" for the poor have been largely pursued in urban slums, but they probably have important implications for rural areas as well. Private group practice clinics, it may be noted, involve a higher percentage of the total physicians in rural counties than in urban, and one can anticipate a wider role for such clinics in the future.

Transportation and communication

A critical aspect of rural health service is the availablity of transportation and communication. It is likely that greater benefits have been brought about in rural health care through improved transportation than through enlargement of medical resources in the isolated rural districts.

Most fundamental are paved roads, which, of course, serve the general marketing needs of agriculture as well as health services. It is ironic that in various countries of Southeast Asia it took the contingencies of guerrilla warfare to produce a network of roads that were long needed anyway for the welfare of rural people; those roads can fortunately facilitate movement of village people to the cities for medical care. On the roads are buses and occasionally taxis for seriously sick patients. Ambulances are also attached to most of the district rural hospitals in Latin America and Asia.

The mobile clinic is widely used in the developing countries as a way of reaching villages distant from a health center. In Malaysia the hospital assistant makes the rounds of several villages once or twice a month, traveling in a small truck that carries a supply of the common drugs. Latin American mobile clinics usually include a physician along with a nursing assistant. In Africa rivers are sometimes used as channels for mobile clinics. A certain romanticism attaches to these patterns, but one must realize that a permanent health post, with an auxiliary worker, is nearly always preferable; a medical consultant can then come by periodically.

Home calls by the physician are becoming rare in most countries, as the demands on the physician's time have increased. The public health nurse or home visitor is more often sent to investigate matters in rural districts. Yet in Great Britain the general practitioner is often proud of his or her continued willingness to make home calls and thereby become acquainted with the real living conditions of the patient. In Belgium the social insurance program pays the country physician not only for the mileage involved in home calls, but also for the time consumed in travel, over and above the fee for the medical service.

For extremely isolated rural people the airplane ambulance is another important adjustment. In Saskatchewan, Canada, when many roads are blocked by snow through the long winter, the airplanes of the Provincial Health Department, notified by telephone or radio, pick up patients and transport them to the main cities; many a nighttime landing has been made on a snow-covered wheat field, illuminated by the headlights of three or four automobiles placed to mark out a runway. The stretches of Siberia have long been served also by airplane ambulances, and in Poland helicopters are used. Australia has its Royal Flying Doctor Service, which is a voluntary agency aided by government grants. More reliance is placed on radiocommunication and transport of the patient nowadays than on conveyance of the physician. Communication by television is the latest adjustment to rural health care problems; the patient's picture is televised to an urban consultant who then advises a general practitioner in the field what should be done. This is now being done between Seattle, Washington and Alaska.

Quality promotion and maintenance

The isolation of rural health workers along with the poverty of rural resources makes it difficult for them to keep up with advances in medical science. Everywhere this problem has been tackled through the principle of regionalization, under which small peripheral rural facilities come under the influence of large urban units.

Regionalization of services is the model for the rural areas of India, Indonesia, Brazil, Sweden, Soviet Union, People's Republic of China, and almost everywhere. The more difficult cases are sent from the peripheral facilities into the central ones, and supervision emanates from the centers outwardly. Rural health personnel may be brought into the main city for various courses of training. Medical schools, of course, along with other types of professional schools bear a special responsibility for such continuing education. Sending medical students out to work with rural physicians is not only valuable for the student but also helps to keep practitioners on their toes.

In the United States the regionalization idea got its first major boost with the Hill-Burton hospital construction program, mentioned earlier. But it took the Regional Medical Program for Heart Disease, Cancer, and Stroke to extend the idea to a functional level. Except for the recent major cutbacks in federal RMP funds, this program was helping to extend the qualitative influence of urban medical centers to rural localities.

Economic support

Basic to the solution of rural health care problems everywhere is attaining adequate economic support. In many countries the social insurance device has strengthened the economic base of medical care in the cities, where insured wage earners live. But most agricultural populations are not brought under the social insurance or social security umbrella for reasons that are economic, administrative, and political. As a result, rural health services have more often depended on support from general national revenues.

In the Scandinavian countries district physicians are supported in the rural areas by the central government, even though they may also earn fees from the health insurance program. The operating costs of health centers and rural hospitals in the developing countries are met typically from national revenues. In the United States the special comprehensive health care programs for American Indians, a largely rural people, are financed by the federal government. The same applies to special family health clinics for migratory or seasonal agricultural workers; formerly all federal, these are now supported by federal grants to the states. In Yugoslavia and Poland small farmers form health cooperatives for meeting both construction and operational costs of certain rural health centers.

So long as the economic base of rural medical care depends solely on rural people, deficiencies must persist; agriculture simply has lower per capita productivity than industry with its greater use of machine power and technology. Rural health care can reach the level of urban health care only by tapping urban wealth. In most countries this is done through use of various types of general revenue. The United States today is debating the issure of national health insurance, as a means of greatly extending economic support for the whole population. We know that voluntary health insurance protection is weakest among rural people, so that there is no doubt that rural people would be the greatest beneficiaries of such a nationwide a program. With such economic underpinning, one could begin to have hope of getting improvements in the health personnel, facilities, and programs that rural areas need.

Health service planning and coordination

The cities, in a sense, can take care of themselves medically, even though there may be extravagance in the use of resources. But for improvement in rural health care, planning is always needed at a national or regional level. This has been recognized in India, in almost all the countries of Africa, in most Latin American countries, and throughout the socialist world.

Health planning has come somewhat later to the industrialized countries of Western Europe and North America, where free private enterprise has been so strong. Yet in America today comprehensive health planning has been launched in all the states, as a result of the federal grants of 1966 for this purpose. So far, the comprehensive health planning programs have accomplished little, but we all know that this is because they have no real authority and very little money. The current period, in my view, is a prelude to planning—a tooling-up period. The action will not really begin until we have a program of nationwide economic support for health services, which will provide the wherewithal and, at the same time, the visible urgency to see that the money is wisely spent.

These eight approaches to solving rural health care problems around the world will doubtless sound familiar. There are very few, among the many specific actions, that have not already been tried somewhere in the United

States, though not always with adequate intensity. In West Virginia with its history of health insurance plans in the mining industry (from the old wage checkoff to the modern Mine Workers' Trust Fund program), its especially strong program of vocational rehabilitation services, its rural hospital construction program, its impressive new school of medicine, and its recent legislation on new forms of paramedical personnel, I suspect that the efforts have been more positive than in most states.

However, as can be seen everywhere, the ultimate solution to rural health care problems is not to be found solely within the borders of rural states or provinces. It demands action on a national level both for mobilization of economic support and for allocation of resources in some proportion to need. Along with these moves, which obviously require governmental initiative, people within a state can organize existing manpower and institutions to be better prepared for national developments. Today we see, for example, the clear invitation from Washington to set up health maintenance organizations as a sound way to systematize both the financing and delivery of health care. We also see many hints at forthcoming expanded support for training new types of health manpower. These steps will strengthen the groundwork for a national health insurance program, which is sure to come in the next few years. With this, the prospects of improving rural health services should become brighter than ever before.

Epilogue

In the last few years, since the papers in the previous chapters were written, there has been continued ferment in the American health services scene, much of it relevant to rural areas. Some of the highlights of this ferment should be noted.

In late 1972 federal amendments to the Social Security Act mandated the establishment of "professional standard review organizations" (PSRO's) to blanket the nation with medical bodies that would exercise peer review of all hospital cases under Medicare and Medicaid. This legislation generated a storm of controversy from the private medical profession, with allegations of government interference in the physician-patient relationship, inhibition of innovative practices in favor of "cookbook medicine," etc. Nevertheless, the surveillance program, which is not really very different from that practiced by diligent governmental and voluntary health insurance programs in the past, gradually got under way. When these PSRO's, some 200 in all, become fully implemented, they should have special significance for monitoring the quality of inpatient work done by the more frequently isolated rural physician. It is generally believed that, in time, the same sort of peer review will be applied to the management of all cases under a national health insurance program, both inside and outside hospitals.

The promotion of health maintenance organizations (HMO's) without specific legislative mandate was discussed in Chapter 1. After extended debate in December 1973 the federal Health Maintenance Organization Act (P.L. 93-222) was enacted in December 1973. This authorized the appropriation of $375,000,000 over a 5-year period for stimulating and assisting in the establishment of new HMO's, with special priorities assigned to coverage of populations in "nonmetropolitan areas." Because of the lesser utilization of health services by rural people, as a result of geographical difficulties, lesser education, and perhaps certain more or less stoical attitudes, the fee-for-service method of medical remuneration is not so lucrative for rural physicians as for urban physicians. Therefore, the HMO concept, with its fixed capitation payments to assure responsibility for the health of an enrolled population, regardless of the volume of services sought or rendered, would have particular advantages for physicians in rural areas. This is quite aside from the incentives inherent in HMO's to promote preventive medicine, make prudent use of costly hospitalization, and generally to attempt to maintain the health of the HMO members.

The movement of the 1960's to establish "neighborhood health centers" for the poor, referred to in several chapters, continued to grow and take on new forms in the 1970's. In 1973 and 1974 all of the health centers for general ambulatory care started by the U.S. Office of Economic Opportunity were transferred to the responsiblity of the Department of Health, Education and Welfare. In addition, a variety of further types of ambulatory care center were established in both urban and rural areas. Under the label of "family health centers," the support for some of these units was shifted from straight federal grants to local prepayment mechanisms both for beneficiaries of Medicaid and Medicare and for self-supporting persons who might be entitled to fringe benefits through labor-management contracts. Health departments, moreover, were beginning to convert their categorical clinics (for child health, venereal disease control, etc.) into generalized ambulatory care centers. While this movement had more vitality in the large cities than the rural districts, there could be no doubt that the general trend in America was toward organization of the delivery of ambulatory service, through a variety of agency-sponsored programs as well as through private group medical practices. By 1970, some 20% of the nation's physicians in clinical work were engaged in group practices, and, as we have noted, this pattern was indeed relatively more prevalent in rural regions.

As of this writing, the wide spectrum of federal bills for national health insurance (NHI) continued to be debated. By late 1974, especially after the swing to the left of the November elections, there was widespread opinion that legislation would soon pass covering all or nearly all the American population with a wider range of benefits than the voluntary insurance movement had made customary. Unsettled were questions such as provisions for cost-sharing by the patient, the role of local insurance agencies as carriers, or intermediaries, or not at all, the exact scope of benefits and population coverage, and the scheme of administration. Under any formula, however, the benefits for rural people would be substantial. Insofar as economic support determines the distribution of health manpower and accessibility to health services, the NHI movement was laying the groundwork for crucial changes in the nationwide distribution of health services.

Finally, with the expiration of legislative authority for the comprehensive health planning (CHP) and regional medical program for various chronic diseases (RMP) programs in 1975, legislation (PL 93-641) was enacted to establish a new network of "health system agencies" (HSA's), which would take over the functions of CHP and RMP and other responsibilities as well. These HSA's would have particular significance for rural areas, in that their delineation would typically include both urban and rural territory, in order to permit a full range of health services to be available within the borders of each area. With a population range of 500,000 to 3,000,000 and averaging about 1,000,000 each, the HSA would provide a practical basis for planning health resources, consultation, and regulation of health services.

These are only the highlights of the health service ferment, as seen in the setting of 1975. The net meaning of it all was a movement, seen worldwide, for an increasing organization of health services—not for the aggrandizement of bureaucracy as such (although some viewed it that way) but as the only path by which greater equity in the distribution of health services in relation to the needs of people, rich and poor, urban and rural, could be attained.